MARKETING STRATEGIES

FOR PHYSICIANS

A GUIDE TO
PRACTICE
GROWTH

MARKETING STRATEGIES

FOR PHYSICIANS

A GUIDE TO PRACTICE GROWTH

STEPHEN W. BROWN, PhD
ANDREW P. MORLEY Jr., MD

MEDICAL ECONOMICS BOOKS
Oradell, NJ 07649

Library of Congress Cataloging-in-Publication Data

Morley, Andrew P.
    Marketing strategies for physicians.

    Includes index.
        1. Medicine—Practice.   2. Medical care—Marketing.
I. Brown, Stephen Walter, 1943-   II. Title.
[DNLM: 1. Marketing of Health Services.   2. Practice
Management, Medical.   W   80   M864m]
R728.M66   1985   610.69'52'0688   85-15436
ISBN 0-87489-405-0

Art Director: Penina M. Wissner
Cover Design: Susan Ahlman & Penina M. Wissner
Cover Photograph: H. Armstrong Roberts, Inc.
Interior Design: Delgado Design Inc.

ISBN 0-87489-405-0

Medical Economics Company Inc.
Oradell, New Jersey 07649

Printed in the United States of America

To Millie Brown
and to
Debbie, Chris, and Blake Morley

CONTENTS

PART III

YOUR MARKETING PLANS
AND PROGRAMS

PART IV

MARKETING APPLICATIONS AND TRENDS

APPENDIX

PREFACE

Future medical historians will be able to characterize the decade of the 1980s with just three words. The first two will be *uncertainty* and *competition*. The third will be today's controversial *marketing*.

For some of you, the term "medical marketing" undoubtedly carries a number of negative connotations—"commercialism," "unprofessionalism," "advertising," and perhaps, even "hucksterism." For others among you, it just as undoubtedly connotes the other extreme—"quick fix" and "panacea." In reality, "medical marketing" is none of the above.

As presented in this book, and as bound by the precepts of its own professional discipline, marketing is an ethical and logical means to develop your practice, a desirable objective in these increasingly competitive times. Moreover, by fully adopting the approach to medicine described in this book, you'll actually be enhancing the quality of care that you provide.

That can happen because marketing focuses on creating a win-win situation that benefits you and the users of the services you provide—patients, other physicians, employers, HMOs, PPOs, and IPAs. Marketing enables you to infuse your practice with a systematic business approach, and imbues you and your staff with a much higher level of sensitivity to patients.

This book was written for the practicing physician. The content is pragmatic and is replete with examples of practices that are successfully using professional marketing techniques. The topics range from developing new clinical services to promotion, and from making yourself more accessible to patients to pricing your services. Of particular interest are the appendices. They provide the sample forms you can use to conduct your personal, professional, and practice assessments, patient surveys, and demographic/competitive analyses.

Others in the health-care industry will also find this book of interest and value. Hospital executives, and their senior managers in areas of planning, marketing, public relations, and physician relations will benefit from its insights, as will department heads and nurses responsible for marketing specific programs that encompass physician involvement. Managers of health plans, dentists, nurses, and other health-care providers will also be able to use the information to practical advantage.

The approach taken in this book is a melding of our respective professional backgrounds and of our work together over the past four years conducting medical marketing seminars and workshops, and consulting with practicing physicians. In a real sense, this book is the synergistic result of those years of our working and learning together. The professional marketer has benefited from the medical orientation of his practicing physician co-author, just as the physician has benefited from the marketing orientation of his marketer co-author.

That process of mutual growth has enabled us to bring medicine and marketing together in a comprehensive approach and methodology designed to help you meet today's competitive challenges. It's called *Marketing Strategies for Physicians.*

Stephen W. Brown, PhD
Tempe, Arizona

Andrew P. Morley, Jr., MD
Decatur, Georgia

ABOUT THE AUTHORS

Individually and jointly over the past four years, the authors have been conducting medical marketing seminars and workshops, serving as consultants for solo and group practices, hospitals, and health systems, and as advisers to a number of organizations, including the American Academy of Family Physicians, the American Express Health Care Faculty, the Lutheran Hospitals and Homes Society, and the Columbia Broadcasting System.

Stephen W. Brown, PhD, is professor of marketing, and director of the First Interstate Center for Services Marketing, Arizona State University, Tempe; 1984-85 president of the 42,000-member American Marketing Association; and a member of the boards of directors of the Academy for Health Services Marketing, Camelback Hospitals, Inc., and The Mahoney Group.

Dr. Brown, who specializes in marketing strategy planning and research, is the author of three other books on marketing, and the author or co-author of more than 80 articles that have appeared in various marketing journals. He serves on the editorial boards of six professional publications, including the *Journal of Health Care Marketing, Physician's Marketing,* and the *Journal of Marketing.*

Andrew P. Morley, Jr., MD, who practices in a five-member family practice group in Decatur, Georgia, is 1984-85 president of the Georgia Academy of Family Physicians, past chairman of the Academy's Public Relations Committee, and past chairman of the Public Relations Committee and the Marketing Advisory Subcommittee of the American Academy of Family Physicians.

Dr. Morley is president of Health Services Marketing, a comprehensive marketing firm for health professionals. He serves as medical editor for the Georgia Radio News Service, and as medical commentator for WXIA-TV, the NBC affiliate in Atlanta. He is the author of many clinical and medical marketing articles, and a member of the editorial boards of the *Journal of the Georgia Academy of Family Physicians* and *Physician's Marketing.*

ACKNOWLEDGMENTS

As with any undertaking of this magnitude, this book was made possible by the efforts and cooperation of many fine people.

Overall, we recognize the imprint on this work of our many colleagues at Arizona State University, the Decatur Clinic, the American Academy of Family Physicians, and the Georgia Academy of Family Physicians.

Special mention to individuals within those organizations must go to Bruce J. Walker, PhD, and Steven D. Wood, PhD (at ASU), and William Myers and William DeLay (at the AAFP). We have also benefited from our professional relationships with Sheryl Bronkesh, MBA, and Camille Day. The diligent assistance of Beth Richards and Sandra Sawyer was invaluable in bringing this book to completion.

We owe special appreciation to Richard Ballad of *Medical Economics* magazine, and to Barbara Pritchard, Reuben Barr, Thomas Bentz, and the staff of Medical Economics Books.

Most important, we give heartfelt thanks to our families for their love and encouragement.

THE CHANGING MEDICAL ENVIRONMENT

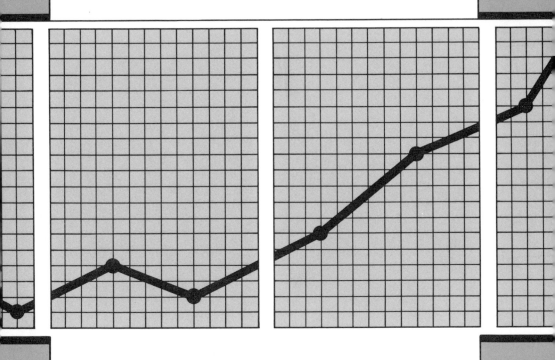

CHAPTER 1

What's happening to our profession?

The practice of medicine is changing—radically. That became quite clear in a conversation between two doctors we know. The older man was lamenting after a long night on call. His colleague, just out of residency, was listening, eager to absorb the wisdom of the ages.

"You know," the senior sighed, "medicine seemed so simple when I started to practice 30 years ago. All I had to worry about was taking care of my patients. Now I have to fret about malpractice, DRGs, HMOs, third-party payers, stiffer competition. Even my patients are changing. They challenge my judgment, tell me they heard differently on the Phil Donahue Show, and God knows what else."

The young doctor thought for a moment, then asked wistfully, "Yeah, there really *was* a time when you didn't have to worry about all that, wasn't there? That must have been paradise."

In many respects, it does seem like paradise lost for both physicians and patients. In the 1950s, the practice of medicine *was* much simpler. The 200,000 physicians who then made up our

3

ranks led much less complicated lives. So did most patients. Seventy-five percent of all doctors were in solo, self-employed practice. Their average net income, before taxes, was around $16,000. Although the cost of starting a practice was the then seemingly outrageous sum of about $10,000, doctors could begin repaying their educational debts within a few months after starting practice.

There was no Medicare, no Medicaid. There were no health maintenance organizations, no preferred provider organizations. The physician's income came almost entirely from cash payments (remember those?) and/or from Blue Shield or some other private insurer; but that was about it. Then the profession began to change rapidly, and a startlingly different medical environment began to emerge, one you must now keep in step with if you're to survive professionally.

The essential fact is that *you must learn to market your services.* That's not an easy idea to accept. Not only the old timers, but many of the more idealistic young physicians are afraid this will mean the end of self-respect, and the end of respect from their communities.

As one young resident said plaintively, "God, I dreamed of becoming a doctor since I was a kid. I went through all that training. Now are you telling me I've got to go out and sell my knowledge and skills as if I were trying to unload a warehouse full of home appliances?"

The answer is No. You don't have to do that, although some do, just as there are lawyers advertising on TV, enticing the public to come forth and sue doctors for malpractice. Quacks and ambulance chasers have always existed in both medicine and law. But they never have, and likely never will, predominate.

Done with taste and discretion, marketing is as honorable as medicine. It can and should force you to become externally oriented—to be aware of changes in competition, government, and patients. You

Figure 1-A
CHANGES IN MEDICAL ENVIRONMENT

Internal Changes	External Changes
• Technology	• Entrepreneurship
• Specialization	• "Big Business"
• Physician Oversupply	• Union Demands
	• Alternative Delivery Systems
	• Government "Quick-Fix" Plans
	• Hospital Re-Orientation
	• Allied Professionals
	• Physician Behavior

must then respond to those challenges in a manner that will both improve your practice while maintaining the highest level of health care. *(See Fig. 1-A)*

You can no longer afford the luxury of nostalgia for the profession's old, internally oriented world—that safe, pleasant, insulated world that was unaffected by the turmoil of the marketplace.

The march of social, economic, and political events is forcing you to participate in the marketing process, or give up medicine. Without marketing expertise, the doctors of tomorrow will survive only if they are wealthy enough to treat their profession as a hobby from which they have no need to make a living. Only the children of the wealthy will be able to afford to practice in the old way.

INTERNAL CHANGES
IN MEDICINE
Today's medicine has been shaped by rapid advances in scientific technology. The change began with the discovery of insulin in 1921. Then a substance was extracted from the liver and used to treat pernicious anemia. In the 1930s, the field of pharmacology was limited to a few special drugs: tincture of digitalis, strychnine, Fowler's solution, and potassium iodide. Penicillin and the sulfa drugs came just before World War II. Since then, thousands of new drugs have become available. Simply keeping up with a few in each classification is a mammoth task.

In diagnostic medicine, the tools of the 1930s were extremely limited. Doctors had the plain roentgenogram, the electrocardiogram, aerobic bacteriology, and a few blood tests. But today, medical technology is limited only by our imagination. CT scans, digital angiography, thallium-cardiac scans, and other space-age advances have rocketed a once rather simple profession into an age of sophistication where the most unbelievable fantasies are realized. And these changes have taken place within the life spans of many physicians practicing today.

Dr. Lewis Thomas, one of the most literate physicians of our day, has commented at length—and in more or less perpetual wonder—at the contrast between the high-tech, high-drama medical and surgical "miracles" that he encounters almost daily at the prestigious New York Hospital, and the simple world of his doctor-father, where perhaps the most important things a physician could bring his patients were faith, warmth, strength, calm, and good humor. Those were almost all the doctor had because his technical armamentarium was virtually bare.

Today, more than one of the doctors who remember that era must pause to ask, "How did it happen? How did it all change?" It had to change, of course. Had it not, millions of lives would have been lost or damaged every year by tuberculosis, polio, and common infections. But the old-timers fear, and quite rightly, that the new technology has some of the elements of the Faustian legend. They don't want to gain spectacular victories if it means losing their souls in the process. And that carries over into a fear and sometimes even loathing of the need to resort to marketing to survive.

Specialization

The technological miracles brought with them the necessity to specialize. There is now too much to learn, too much to know to allow anyone to claim mastery over the whole body of medical knowledge. There is little room for Renaissance men or women in a world where the production, processing, and communication of information is rapidly becoming a leading industry.

Back in the 1930s, a doctor could justly claim that he knew most of what there was to know about medicine. As we've noted, his lack of extensive tools with which to heal the sick led him to develop his personality, his bedside manner, and his ability to psychically affect the welfare of his patient.

As a result, the doctor was, in many ways, more respected than he is today. Possibly a part of this was that "doctor" was still a relatively rare term, since we had not yet spawned the vast hordes of PhDs that now complicate the use of the title doctor.

In those days, doctors were general practitioners, surgeons, or internists. And the only subspecialty areas of internal medicine were in dermatology, neurology, and tuberculosis. As clinical manifestations of myocardial infarctions were recognized, cardiology was born. There were also respectable advances in microbiology and physiology, and the fields of endocrinology and pulmonary medicine took shape. But when World War II broke out, only 25 percent of all doctors were specialists. Today it's close to 60 percent.

In area after area the profession subdivided like some mad amoeba. By 1950, many physicians began to feel that they *had* to become subspecialists or risk extinction, drowned in the flood of new information and new technology.

Today, this is backfiring on us. Compared with just a decade ago, we have approximately 50 percent more neurologists, 60 percent more cardiologists, and 120 percent more gastroenterologists. This has helped create an environment of stepped-up competition. One example: The older doctor in our opening scene is a general internist who no longer sees heart attack or ulcer patients. They go to the subspecialists.

The number of surgeons has increased so much—from 67,000 in 1970 to 84,000 in 1980—that many general surgeons are finding it hard to keep privileges in subspecialty areas. Frustration is rampant. Yet, though specialists outnumber primary-care doctors, about half of all patient encounters are still in primary care.

Specialists are now doing a lot of primary care work because they're finding it hard to make a living from patients in their specialty areas.

A surgeon friend actively solicits patients to come to him for their general health needs. As he put it, "That's better than having to take a second job in the emergency room to get my kids through college."

In a recent physician survey conducted by the AMA, 73 percent of the respondents said there is a surplus of specialists, especially in surgery and internal medicine.

Physician Oversupply

In 1958, the number of students graduated from America's then 85 medical schools was 6,861. Though the ratio was only 144 physicians per 100,000 population, concern over competition was already growing.

Today there are 127 medical schools—almost a 50 percent increase in 27 years—turning out a potential graduating class of 16,000 doctors every year. By 1980, the doctor-patient ratio had increased to more than 200 per 100,000 of population. To put it another way: While our general population is growing at 0.86 percent per year, the physician population is increasing by 2.8 percent—or three times as fast. *(See Fig. 1-B)*

Figure 1-B
PHYSICIAN-TO-POPULATION RATIO

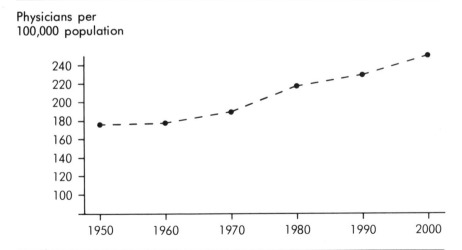

Physicians per
100,000 population

Figure 1-C
PHYSICIAN SUPPLY AND REQUIREMENTS FOR 1990

	Physicians	Total Residents	Total Supply	Require- ments	Surplus (Shortage)
All Physicians	504,750	88,500	535,750	466,000	69,750
General/Family Practice	84,800	9,900	88,250	84,000	4,250
General Pediatricians	35,300	7,050	37,750	30,250	7,500
Pediatric Allergy	750	450	900	900	—
Pediatric Cardiology	850	400	1,000	1,150	(150)
Pediatric Endocrinology	250	0	250	800	(550)
Pediatric Hematology-Oncology	500	200	550	1,650	(1,100)
Pediatric Nephrology	200	50	200	350	(150)
Neonatology	700	—	700	1,300	(600)
General Internal Medicine	66,500	20,800	73,800	70,250	3,550
Allergy and Immunology	3,000	150	3,050	2,050	1,000
Cardiology	14,250	1,900	14,900	7,750	7,150
Endocrinology	3,700	500	3,850	2,050	1,800
Gastroenterology	6,550	1,000	6,900	6,500	400
Hematology-Oncology	7,850	1,300	8,300	9,000	(700)
Infectious Diseases	3,050	500	3,250	2,250	1,000
Nephrology	4,600	700	4,850	2,750	2,100
Pulmonary Diseases	6,600	1,050	6,950	3,600	3,350
Rheumatology	2,850	500	3,000	1,700	1,300
Neurology*	8,300	950	8,650	5,500	3,150
Dermatology	7,150	700	7,350	6,950	400
Psychiatry (General)	29,250	2,550	30,500	38,500	(8,000)
Child Psychiatry	4,050	200	4,100	9,000	(4,900)
Obstetrics-Gynecology	32,300	6,200	34,450	24,000	10,450
General Surgery	32,100	9,200	35,300	23,500	11,800
Neurosurgery	4,850	700	5,100	2,650	2,450
Ophthalmology	15,400	2,600	16,300	11,600	4,700
Orthopedic Surgery	19,000	3,150	20,100	15,100	5,000
Otolaryngology	8,000	1,400	8,500	8,000	500
Plastic Surgery	3,700	600	3,900	2,700	1,200
Thoracic Surgery	2,700	450	2,900	2,050	850
Urology	8,800	1,600	9,350	7,700	1,650
Emergency Medicine	8,900	1,000	9,250	13,500	(4,250)
Preventive Medicine	5,550	0	5,550	7,300	(1,750)
Anesthesiology*	18,750	2,050	19,450	21,000	(1,550)
Nuclear Medicine*	150	0	150	4,000	(3,850)
Pathology*	16,000	2,450	16,850	13,500	3,350
Physiatry*	2,350	150	2,400	3,200	(800)
Radiology*	26,450	3,800	27,800	18,000	9,800
All other and unspecified	9,200	1,450	9,700	—	N/A

*Source: Graduate Medical Education National Advisory Council Reprinted from October 3, 1980 AMA News

The now famous 1980 report of the Graduate Medical Educational National Advisory Committee (GMENAC) predicted that if medical schools continue to graduate classes of the present size, there will be a half million doctors in this country by 1990, an oversupply of about 70,000. The only areas in which there won't be a surplus, according to the report, are pediatrics, hematology, psychiatry, and emergency medicine. *(See Fig. 1-C)*

Many specialty organizations have discussed the validity of the findings, and most agree that the MD side of the physician-to-patient ratio will continue to rise.

If these predictions are not sobering enough, the number of foreign medical graduates (FMGs) is expected to increase by 40,000 to 50,000 over the next 10 years—a staggering addition to an already engorged physician force. The result can only be a more competitive environment, and this, inescapably, leads back to the fact that physicians must develop an understanding of, and an appreciation for, the professional marketing of their services.

EXTERNAL PRESSURES
ON THE PROFESSION

The competitive environment in the profession of medicine is also being created by external forces. These pressures are applied by other professionals, big business, government, new means of delivering care, shrinking markets, and rising costs.

Allied Professionals

Paralleling the growing number of physicians is the alarming rate of increase in the supply of nurses, physical therapists, and other health-care deliverers. In 1960, there were only four allied professionals for every physician. By 1970, there were eight. By 1980, there were 20. This doesn't mean there isn't an important place for these people, but it's another indication of the increasing complexity and competition within the health-delivery system.

The GEMNAC report projected that by 1990 there will be more than 30,000 nurse practitioners and more than 20,000 physicians' assistants. This would be acceptable except that many of them are seeking the legal right to practice medicine, and an increasing number of state legislators are becoming sympathetic to their wishes. To add this potential new group of health-care providers to the projected surplus of physicians would change the issue from a problem into a disaster for doctors.

Competing Physicians

No longer can you simply hang out a shingle and expect your reception area to be magically filled with the sick and injured. Highly qualified physicians are finding it difficult to attract enough patients to make ends meet, especially in the first years of practice. With too many doctors in general and too many specialists in particular, with an increasing number of allied health professionals and an army of foreign medical graduates poised for invasion, competition is here to stay.

We recall a conversation with a recent residency graduate in South Carolina. He was filled with enthusiasm about his future:

"I've waited all my life to practice medicine," he said. "Now I can begin to pay off some debts and give my family a few nice things."

But after 18 months he became cynical and discouraged. Just as he began his practice, the community accepted an application for a new emergency center. A year later, many of the established doctors in the area formed an HMO. Our new doctor—wiser about the pitfalls of practice, and acutely aware of his competitive environment—reluctantly moved his family, and his dreams, to another community.

That experience isn't limited to young practitioners. While in the emergency room a few months ago, we spotted a surgeon friend.

"Going to take out an appendix?"

"No," he sighed. "I work here on weekends now."

And this was a really *good* surgeon who'd been in practice many years. But there were 10 new surgeons in the community aggressively seeking new patients, and so his practice had fallen off sharply.

"You know, my son is a senior in college now," he said. "And my daughter begins in the fall. My income seems to be dropping all the time. I just had to find some way to make ends meet until my surgical practice picks up again."

All across the country, physicians are leaving their primary specialty for other areas of endeavor, or moving to other communities, or even abandoning the practice of medicine completely. It used to be that physicians were satisfied with their small piece of the health-care "pie." But that pie is being cut into smaller and smaller slices. Whether physicians realize it or not, the real name for their current struggle to survive is "marketing your services," and too many are floundering, not knowing how to go about it.

The Big Business of Health

The economics of medicine were relatively simple 30 years ago. Office visits were as low as $3 and seldom more than $15, even in high-priced New York City. And most patients paid cash. Some physicians laugh at stories of depression days when doctors got paid in chickens and eggs. There was a time, nevertheless, when the barter system was not only acceptable, but advantageous. A doctor got along very well with one nurse and a receptionist-book-keeper. The office staff spent little time dealing with insurance forms, and insurers usually paid without a hassle.

Somehow, what used to be a small, manageable profession has transformed itself, or has been transformed, into the third largest industry in America—a business that employs some five million people. The Health Care Finance Administration informs us that America's health-care costs climbed to $322.4 billion in 1983, more than 10 percent of the gross national product. As a result, the medical profession is being invaded by an ever-growing number of investors and developers. These health-care entrepreneurs take their cue from Georges Clemenceau, the French statesman, who said that war is much too serious a matter to leave to the generals. Today's business tycoons find it equally difficult to leave this potential trillion-dollar health-care industry in the hands of a bunch of practitioners.

The Corporate Hospital

One of the prime examples of the new entreprenurial system is the evolution of the hospital. Many are no longer owned and operated by the communities in which they're located. All over the nation, large conglomerates are taking over or are creating chains of hundreds of hospitals. The Hospital Corporation of America is the largest for-profit, health-care provider with more than 400 well-equipped, computerized hospitals. The shares of this multi-million-dollar corporation are traded on Wall Street. By 1990, at least half of the nation's hospitals will be owned by such private corporations. Why has big business gotten so deeply into the business of health? Well, there happen to be at least 118 billion reasons—all of them dollars.

As far as most physicians are concerned, however, the major change in the role of the hospital has been its entry into primary care. The change came because people came to use emergency rooms as a community service. When the number of hospital out-patient visits quadrupled between 1965 and 1976, it became obvious that people were using the emergency room because they had no alternative.

The hospitals' marketing specialists felt a need was being demonstrated that could, and should, be met. The trouble was that the cost of running an ER was growing at an astonishing rate. A cheaper way had to be found. The answer was a primary-care center located on the hospital campus, but operating at a lower cost, with the patient pool to be drawn from the emergency room. More than 3,000 of our country's larger hospitals now have at least one out-patient facility, and some have a number of centers off campus. Hospitals are thus trying to become comprehensive health-care delivery systems rather than a part of the whole, and apparently it's working. Many of them are expanding to include several out-patient services—such as surgery and diagnostic testing—and will continue to do so as long as there are other markets.

In many cases, patients treated by out-patient services are those who might otherwise be visiting private practitioners. The delivery of health care within a hospital setting is growing so rapidly that one out of every 12 primary-care physicians works full time for a hospital.

Recently a rural Midwestern physician told us, with some agitation, that her hospital had opened an emergency room.

"It didn't affect me at first," she said. "But then they began to see more and more patients who were not really emergencies. Then they actually began to solicit patients to come in for immunizations and camp physicals, and other routine care. Now they've spread out in the community. They're taking my patients away from me!" Once her ally, the hospital has become her adversary. Her final comment showed her frustration.

"What can I do about it?" she asked. "They have big bucks behind them. I can't compete with that kind of money." (Actually, she could and did compete, when she was shown how.)

So, the fact must be accepted that many hospitals are now actually "practicing medicine," and are often in direct competition with private practitioners.

Freestanding Treatment Centers

Spreading speedily across the country, operating under a variety of names and fiscal arrangements, these convenient medical centers operate in response to the need for a more economical and convenient way to receive "emergency" care.

The medical establishment has quite rightly attacked many of these facilities as not being true "emergency rooms." But for the most part, that argument doesn't dissuade the public from using them. More than 20 million people already have visited freestanding clinics. That's not bad for an idea that wasn't born until the early 1970s.

Investment analysts predict that these centers could attract as much as 25 percent of the nearly $50 billion that Americans spend annually on out-patient services. That means these business ventures in the medical field could reap higher profits than the fast-foods industry. Small wonder they are being dubbed, "Medical McDonald's" or "McDoc's."

Is it just a fad that will go as quickly as it came? The National Association for Ambulatory Care (NAFAC) doesn't think so. It estimates that as many as 2,600 centers already were in operation in July 1985, and that new ones are opening at a rate of one a day.

Who are these entrepreneurs who are attracting all the patients? Well, the vast majority of the centers are leased, owned, and/or operated by *physicians*—reputable men and women who saw a need and met it. They are, in short, *marketing* their services. And why not?

These centers grew out of a need patients have been expressing for years to doctors who didn't listen. When patients began turning to emergency rooms to avoid the long waits for appointments with their private physicians, most doctors didn't really care. They were busy enough and felt the patients would eventually return. But when the emergency rooms became overcrowded, the patients didn't go back to the private practitioners. They found an alternative in the freestanding medical centers—and they're still going to them by the millions. The market automatically provided an answer to the question of customer convenience while most physicians remained silent.

Government Intervention

As we all know, the federal government certainly hasn't remained silent during the recent history of medicine. As early as 1957, Congress was discussing the Forand Bill, a proposal to cover hospital costs for the aged on Social Security. But because of the projected annual cost—a then enormous sum of $2 billion—the bill was soundly defeated. Yet, Congress finally took an active role. Of the many changes in this country's health-care system, perhaps none is as significant as the introduction by Congress of Medicare. Signed into law on July 30, 1965, this legislation changed the practice of medicine forever.

Originally designed to help care for the elderly, Medicare was later joined by Medicaid, the plan for the health care of all the needy. The medical profession vigorously opposed this legislation. But the American public demanded it. Unfortunately, the question of how to pay for it was left in a somewhat cloudy state.

Diagnosis Related Groupings (DRG) is the government's attempt at a quick-fix scheme to curb rising costs. It requires that payments to hospitals be based on diagnosis, rather than length of stay and collective expenses. This newest "alphabet" registration has placed untold stress on hospitals and physicians. But DRG—or some variant—is here to stay.

Rising Costs _____ Equally important changes have been taking place in the labor movement and in employee benefits. Many years ago, the only people concerned with the cost of health care were the patients who were paying, the doctors who were collecting, and the insurance carriers who footed the bill. But when medical care became a large part of labor's demands, the unions became strong advocates for lowering the cost of health care. And one sleeping giant awoke another when big business found itself having to pay for these new employee benefits. Changes became inevitable.

Health costs now represent the fastest growing expense of doing business in America. For instance, the price of every Ford automobile is increased $400 because of employee health-care costs.

These rising costs helped encourage the emergence of non-traditional providers—such as health maintenance organizations (HMOs), individual practice associations (IPAs), and preferred provider organizations (PPOs). More than 300 HMOs have already enrolled 13 million Americans. These organizations are designed to provide financial incentives for employees to choose physicians and other providers on a cost basis. Although employee insurance options normally don't preclude reimbursement for traditional fee-for-service care, the cost of such care is typically greater than those of HMOs or PPOs.

These new organizations are being encouraged by government. As the nation's largest insurer via Medicare and Medicaid, and as a major funder of other types of health care, governmental bodies are aggressively seeking new ways to cut the costs. Consumers are being encouraged by government to consider the cost-benefit trade-offs associated with health care. Moreover, through DRGs, providers are being urged, if not forced, to be more sensitive to costs.

Figure 1-D
EXTERNAL COMPETITIVE ENVIRONMENT
_____

- Entrepreneurs
- Large-Group Practices
- Pre-Paid Plans
- Hospitals
- Free-Standing Clinics
- Provider Arrogance
_____

Summary
_____ All the changes we've enumerated have brought marketing into prominence among forward-looking physicians. Still, marketing may represent the least understood term in medicine today. The next chapter shows that marketing is far more than selling or advertising. The application of marketing to a practice can represent a "win-win" situation for both patient and physician, and it can actually improve the quality of medical practice.

Resources

Graduate Medical Educational National Advisory Committee Report (1980).
Health Care Finance Administration Report (1984).
National Association of Free-Standing Emergency Centers Report (1983).

CHAPTER 2

Is marketing really a monster?

A lot of physicians, worried about the future, are muttering about marketing. You hear them speaking anxiously—and with some bewilderment—of selling, pricing, HMOs, PPOs, IPAs, PR, advertising, promotion, cost per thousand, and so on. How can all these terms, these intruders from the hard world of commerce, fit into your previously insular world of medicine?

Well, our purpose is to help you break that logjam of misunderstandings. The premise is quite simple: Marketing is nothing more than focusing on the needs and wants of those who use your services—patients, other physicians, referring agencies, and employers—and then developing the programs and services to meet those needs and wants.

This book is the product of the authors' years of involvement in health-services marketing, one of us practicing medicine, and lecturing and consulting, and the other studying, researching, teaching, and consulting, particularly with physicians, in the marketing discipline. Our objective is to help you better understand and utilize marketing, and enhance your practice and personal growth.

We're now going to look at five medical marketing observations that will provide a foundation for the remaining chapters in this book.

A FIVE-POINT MARKET PERSPECTIVE

1. Marketing is viewed and implemented too narrowly by physicians and health-services organizations.
2. Most medical-services marketers have little training or experience in marketing.
3. In the minds of many medical people, negativism and skepticism still surround the practice of marketing.
4. Marketing has been oversimplified and oversold in some health/medical situations.
5. Most importantly, within a practice, marketing is usually not viewed as everyone's business, but just the responsibility of the doctor and/or the office manager.

These observations form a perspective that's both sobering and enlightening. It's sobering because we're beginning to recognize that marketing isn't a panacea or quick fix for all the major challenges facing the health and medical-services organizations. But the observations are also enlightening because they form the foundation for realistic and achievable strategies for your practice. And that's what we try to do for you in this book.

1. THE NARROW VIEW

The most frequent mistake of physicians new to marketing is to see a part for the whole. "Marketing is just advertising," or "Marketing is really nothing but promotion." This stems largely from failing to recognize the multiple "target markets" available and the range of marketing strategies and tactics to consider. For hospitals, the consumer has been primarily the physician and, more recently, also the patient. A more enlightened view would now include employers, third-party payers, the government, other health-related agencies, and the hospital's employees, all as "constituencies," to borrow a political term.

In your practice there are also several categories of constituents. The first, of course, is your patient population. But other physicians are also among your major constituents and are especially vital to the success of subspecialists heavily dependent on referrals. Extending your vision even further, you can see other individuals and groups that may influence your practice, such as employers, government, social-service agencies, third-party payers, and media.

The tendency, however, is to become preoccupied with only one or two components of marketing. To some, marketing is nothing more than glorified public relations, and the person who has been responsible for PR may be given a promotion and/or a new title and be expected to suddenly look and act like a health-services marketer.

It's natural that marketing's most visible components, advertising and promotion, are often mistaken for marketing as a whole. When practices adopt this view and a promotional strategy fails, all the blame falls on promotion. The strategy actually may have been very good, but a misunderstood and narrow perception of marketing may have undercut its effectiveness.[1] So physicians must learn to identify all of marketing's components and use a variety of them in skillful combinations.

In working with many health organizations for the past five years, we've found it helpful to use a framework we call the *marketing umbrella*. A discussion of each of the components embraced under this symbol is beyond the scope of this chapter, but some idea of its far-reaching effects is given in Figure 2-A.

Figure 2-A
COMPONENTS OF THE MARKETING UMBRELLA

- Research and Analysis: Gathering and digesting pertinent information from outside your practice, and assessing its impact, e.g., patient survey, demographics, trends.

- Strategic Planning: Articulating the actions necessary to help realize goals in practice and marketing strategy planning, and identifying priority areas of practice opportunity, e.g., geriatrics, sports medicine, hypertension.

- Product/Service Development, Modification, and Elimination: Infusing a market with new services and modifications, and deleting certain existing services.

- Pricing: Imposing market-based input on fee setting and presenting your prices to users of your services.

- Distribution and Accessibility: Looking from the user's perspective at your practice's services, and developing methods to improve accessibility to them.

- Personal Selling, Advertising, and Public Relations: Informing existing and potential patients of your various services through a variety of modes, e.g., personal discussions, newsletters, community involvement.

- Evaluation and Control: Monitoring your progress.

2. UNDERTRAINED AND INEXPERIENCED MARKETERS

Most of those who have recently emerged as health-care marketers are bright, conscientious, and well-intended. Unfortunately, they usually are novices thrust into this new area with little training or guidance. The new marketers in hospitals often have considerable health-service experience, but in areas such as public relations, planning, or development—not in marketing as a complete discipline. They haven't had extensive marketing courses or the work experiences enjoyed by many practicing marketers in other industries. Among private practitioners the absence of marketing know-how is even more pronounced, and the typical practice often relies on the part-time—and often reluctant—efforts of a physician or office manager. Sometimes these important activities are farmed out to a practice-management consultant or an advertising/PR agency.

This was brought home to us when we were approached by the administrator of a multi-specialty group practice.

"We need to hire a director of marketing," he announced. "But I'm more interested in a marketing person than a health-services type. I'm pessimistic about finding many genuine marketers within a hospital or any other health-organization setting. I'm inclined to hire a good marketer of consumer products or a bank marketer, and then let him or her learn about the medical practice on the job."

The dilemma is widespread. Many health-services organizations are looking outside the industry for personnel as they scramble to become more marketing oriented.

Facing this challenging situation, it obviously behooves the dedicated physician with minimal marketing training or experience to get educated quickly. And while there's no substitute for on-the-job experience, a fair knowledge of marketing can be acquired more swiftly by attending seminars, workshops, and convention sessions offered by such groups as the American Academy of Family Physicians (AAFP), the American Medical Association (AMA), and the American Group Practice Association (AGPA). Reading material supplied by these organizations can also be useful. (See, for example, the AAFP's "Honing the Competitive Edge" kit).

As this book is being written, we're also witnessing the birth of many new physician-marketing newsletters of varying quality. Reading the *Journal of Health Care Marketing* with its fine articles, minicases, resource guide, book/article reviews, and abstracts is another source of knowledge. Other less specialized publications, such as *Medical Economics, The Internist,* and *AAFP Reporter*, feature articles on marketing-related topics.

Attending the annual Symposium of Health Services Marketing, sponsored by the Academy of Health Care Marketing of the American Marketing Association, and reading the books offered by Aspen Systems Corp., are other ways of learning about the more general field of health-care marketing.

If the subject is new to you, we strongly encourage you to increase your knowledge of services marketing in general, and not *just* medical marketing. You can enroll in regular or continuing-education marketing classes at almost any college, since marketing is one of the most popular majors today.

Also, you can join in the activities of the American Marketing Association, and its Academy of Health Care Marketing. Finally, there are many practical periodicals, such as *The Marketing News* (American Marketing Association, 250 South Wacker Drive, Chicago, IL 60606) and *Advertising Age* (Crain Communications Inc., 740 North Rush Street, Chicago, IL 60611), as well as numerous books on the subject. Given all this, we see that marketing has earned the right to be called a major discipline.

3. NEGATIVE IMAGE

Despite the strides marketing has made, and its increasing acceptance within the health care industry, its nature and use can still conjure negative images. It is still regarded as unprofessional and/or unethical in some circles. Even among practices and professions that make use of it, marketing is often viewed somewhat guiltily as a necessary evil, brought about primarily by the perils of increased competition.

Our involvement with the executives of a major national medical association illustrates these suspicious attitudes. One of us is currently retained by this organization as its marketing adviser. But in the initial contact with them, four years ago, they checked us out very carefully. They were as interested in our personal stance and philosophy relative to physician-practice development as they were in our professional expertise in that area.

Doctors certainly don't want to commit themselves to be guided by inexpert or casual advice, and we applaud this "look before we leap" stance—so long as this very necessary leap *is* eventually made.

To a great extent, skeptical attitudes stem from the implications associated with our earlier observations that marketing remains a foggy concept, often equated with its most visible and potentially controversial components: advertising, promotion, and selling.

For these reasons, in our presentations to physicians we address marketing's image problems and misunderstandings up front. We then point out that the implementation of marketing strategies and tactics can't be standardized because it varies not only from industry to industry, but from setting to setting. Even within medicine, what works for a new obstetrical/gynecological practice may be substantially different from what works for a long-standing neurological practitioner.

While it may have been, or still is referred to by some other names—practice development, public relations, development—marketing has been utilized to some extent by doctors and the health-care industry for decades. But now competition and other external forces have suddenly made marketing crucial for everyone in the health profession. Thus, the issue today is not *whether* health and medical providers engage in marketing, but whether they do it *well*.[2,3]

4. OVERSIMPLIFICATION AND OVERSELLING

Marketing has been oversimplified and oversold by too many health-services marketers, and to a lesser extent by top-level, health-services decision makers. This has been compounded by the often narrow and misunderstood view of marketing held by so many of the rank and file in the health care field. Yet, recent challenges—such as alternative delivery systems, modified reimbursement patterns, and changing consumer attitudes—have led many to look to marketing for a quick fix for sagging revenues and deteriorating patient levels.

Marketing is under great pressure to rapidly create and implement new programs and services and new promotional campaigns. Unfortunately, this pressure often results in the hard-pressed marketer giving lip service to a thorough examination of the market opportunity when, out of necessity, he is blindly copying the general pattern used by other providers. Is it any wonder an increasing percentage of new health-care products and services fail each year?

5. MARKETING IS EVERYBODY'S BUSINESS

Nothing we have told you is more important than one fact: Marketing is everyone's business, not just the concern of the physician, the office manager, or someone with the word marketing in his or her job title.[4] Let's look at some examples of why this is true.

Last winter, a neighbor finally gave up trying to overcome a lingering cold on his own. He had no family doctor, so he went to see a Dr. Simpson, recommended to him by his son, who was on the high school basketball team. Dr. Simpson was the team doctor, and the boys liked him. Our neighbor had met him briefly and had been impressed by a presentation the doctor had made at the Rotary Club.

Our neighbor left work early one afternoon and went to the doctor's office. He didn't have an appointment, but he knew Dr. Simpson was just beginning his practice, and was accepting new patients. He went up to the reception window and asked if he could see the doctor. The initial inquiry met with no response from the secretary, who was intently chewing gum and typing.

Our friend then raised his voice and again asked if he could see the doctor. This time the secretary heard him, but continued to type. She did condescend to communicate via a frustrated shrug of one shoulder and the laconic observation, "The doctor's busy, so you have to wait." Given this treatment, the man walked out, never to return.

The young doctor will probably never know that the incident occured. Though he is personally marketing-oriented, he's failed to infuse marketing thinking and behavior in his staff. As a result, his infant practice is being smothered in its cradle.

To instill new ways of thinking and behaving in your employees, you must begin at the top—with yourself. A report by McKinsey & Company, one of the world's most prestigious and pragmatic consulting firms, led to the best-selling book, *In Search of Excellence.*[5] The report reviews the characteristics and unique features of some of America's most successful corporations, such as Hewlett-Packard and McDonald's. A hallmark of most of these firms is a "closeness to the customer" that permeates the organization and all its employees. It's common for many of the top executives to spend a number of days each month in contact with current and potential customers. These experiences help them monitor the ever-changing marketplace while they're implicitly or explicitly selling the customers on the firm's products.

Each of these companies has a marketing department with personnel specializing in research, promotion/advertising, personal selling, distribution, and other activities. Yet, by their actions and words, the top executives are constantly demonstrating that marketing is everyone's business, not just the focus of the marketing department. These companies are "customer driven."

And so it should be in the increasingly competitive medical environment of the 1980s. Starting from the top, all personnel must recognize that the very existence of the practice—and therefore their jobs—depends on their relations with their customers. Medical practices, hospitals, and other organizations in which this appreciation is widespread take on special qualities of consumer sensitivity that ultimately pay off.

CHAPTERS TO COME

So marketing is a discipline in and of itself. Books and articles have been written on general marketing, as well as on specific areas, such as consumer behavior, marketing research, and promotion. Although this book is more general in nature, its major purpose is to take the established resources and expertise of the marketing world and apply them in medical-practice settings.

As a backdrop for the remaining chapters, a conceptual model of physician marketing should be helpful to you. The two major entities are the medical practice itself and the target markets that each practice chooses to feature. Target markets are linked to the practice by formal surveys and informal, word-of-mouth marketing research. The practice's interface with its target markets are through its marketing mix of product/service, pricing, place/accessibility, and promotion/communication. The model also illustrates that government, competition, economics, and other outside influences affect both the marketplace and the practice. *(See Fig. 2-B)*

Chapters 3-6 present directions for self-assessment. You're led through a set of evaluations of your wants, needs, and goals, both personal and professional, and of your practice. Only by understanding yourself and your practice can you determine how to best utilize marketing. There's no single, grand marketing design that works for everyone. The development and implementation of marketing plans vary because every physician and every practice is unique.

Chapter 7 shows how to divide your current and potential patients into target markets, or market segments. Market segmentation will enable you to rethink your current and future patient base by categorizing your patients into various groupings, each of which can be targeted for particular attention.

Beginning with Chapter 8, Part III takes you outside your practice and into the setting of those who use your services. We introduce you to patients—their attitudes and behaviors—in ways you may not have considered. The benefits and methods of marketing research are also discussed with particular attention to patient surveys.

Many of the major "HOW TOs" of the book are found in Chapters 9-14. Chapter 9 lays out the hows and whys of marketing planning. The following chapters focus on the components of your plan, the 4 Ps of the marketing mix: Product/service, Pricing, Place/accessibility, and Promotion/communication. Although each of these elements is already being used by virtually all physicians, the marketing approach focuses on the user's orientation. Chapter 14 traces the key steps to understanding and keeping the patients you've got.

Chapters 15-18 deal with clinical-services marketing applications, an analysis of malpractice dangers, and a projection of medical and

Figure 2-B
MODEL OF PHYSICIAN MARKETING

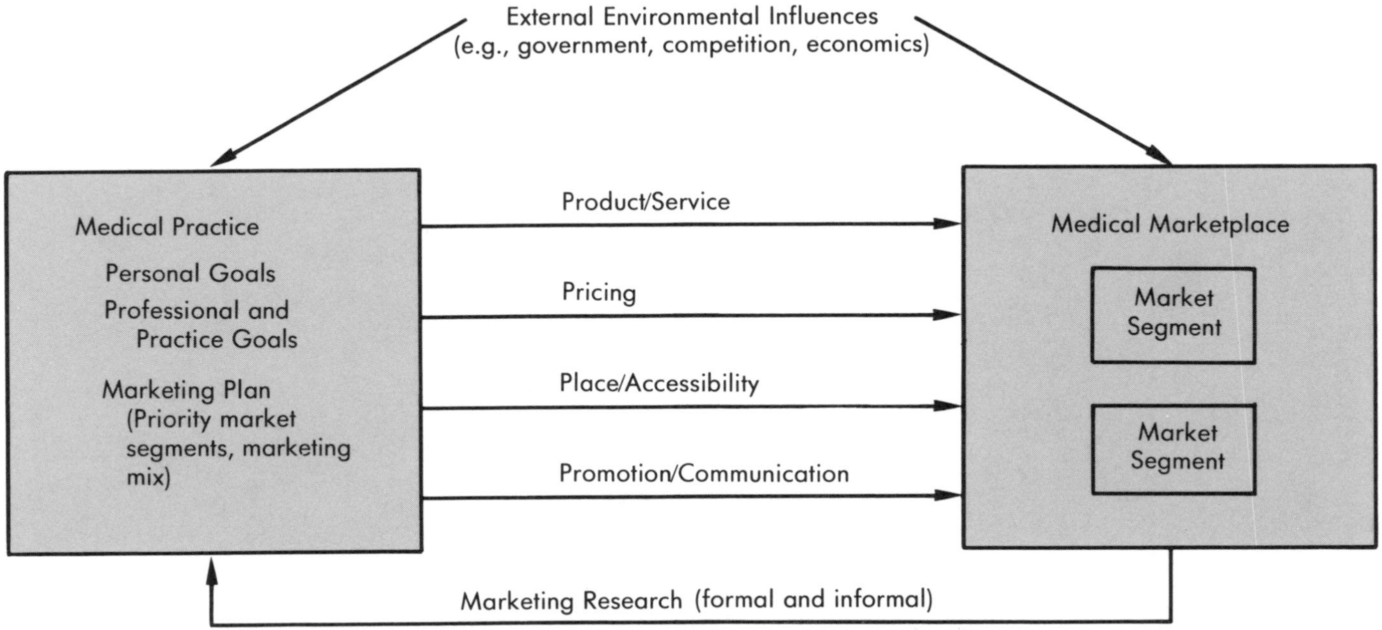

Medical Marketplace

Market Segment

Market Segment

External Environmental Influences
(e.g., government, competition, economics)

Product/Service

Pricing

Place/Accessibility

Promotion/Communication

Marketing Research (formal and informal)

Medical Practice

Personal Goals

Professional and Practice Goals

Marketing Plan
(Priority market segments, marketing mix)

marketing trends. Although not typically thought of in a clinical vein, many of the fundamentals of marketing can be selectively used to better understand and treat patients, to meet their needs and increase their compliance, to improve your practice and reduce the threat of malpractice.

Summary

Despite some of the criticisms and caveats sprinkled throughout this book, the future is bright for marketing medical practices, and for dedicated health-services marketers. The understanding and appreciation of marketing is broadening as well as deepening. Learning experiences coupled with a commitment to marketing education bode well for the maturing of physician marketing, and for the dedicated individuals who have chosen to work in this area.

In addition to these positive developments, all indications point to a health- and medical-services future where marketing becomes necessary for success, and in many cases, for survival. As in all the great challenges of life, the problems facing the medical profession in general also offer great opportunities. All you have to do is seize them.

References

1. Clarke RN: Marketing health care, problems in implementation. *Health Care Management Review*, 3 (Winter 1982), 21-27.
2. Kotler P, Murray M: Third sector management, the role of marketing. *Public Administration Review*. September-October 1975, 476-472.
3. Lamb CW Jr, Finn DW: Has marketing been oversold to hospital administrators? *Journal of Health Care Marketing*, 2 (Fall 1982), 43-46.
4. Brown SW: Candid observations on the status of health services marketing, *Journal of Health Care Marketing*, 3 (Summer 1983), 45-52.
5. Peters TJ, Waterman RH: *In Search of Excellence*, New York: Harper & Row, 1982.

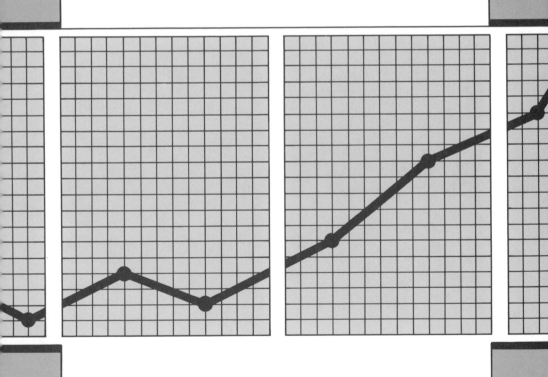

PART II

ANALYZING YOURSELF AND THE MARKETPLACE

CHAPTER 3

What are your goals? How will you reach them?

A physician from the Midwest came to us with a familiar problem; he needed to increase his patient load. He was ready to do anything—except begin at the beginning.

"What are your goals for your practice?" we asked.

"More patients!" he quickly responded.

"Yes, we know, but what do you want from the profession of medicine—*personally?*"

He looked puzzled, and responded with some hesitation, "Besides a better income, I'm not sure."

His fuzziness illustrates one of the major pitfalls of starting a marketing plan: the temptation to begin without any direction or accurate assessment of your true goals.

Before you can develop and implement an effective marketing plan, you have to define what you want, both personally and professionally, from your practice. Would you go into any other business venture without first assessing the expectations of your investment? So why should the marketing of your medical practice be any different?

Let's start by looking at some personal factors that might influence your marketing decisions. We'll follow with an examination of how your professional goals interact with your personal desires. We'll then build on that and tackle the factors involved in formulating your practice goals. *(See Fig. 3-A)*

PERSONAL GOALS

Before you can get a firm grasp on what your personal wants really are, you should take a close look at your time and money needs. The time factor encompasses the years you have left until retirement.

Time

A physician in the Southeast recently began his plan by writing in bold letters, "I MUST TAKE A HALF DAY OFF!" When we asked why he put so much emphasis on that, he said it was extremely important for both his emotional and physical health that he have time to swim. So that had to become part of any marketing plan we suggested. Another doctor was having marital problems and promised his wife that he'd spend more time with his family. So time off had to be an essential part of his plan.

You have to define such personal limitations and needs before you begin. If you don't, whatever you do to improve your practice will end up clashing with your real desires.

Retirement

This is a key time factor. If you're just starting out, your goal will be to build a practice by using a total marketing approach. But if retirement is in your near future, there are marketing plans that offer short-term solutions.

Figure 3-A
ASSESSING YOUR WANTS AND NEEDS

Personal	Professional	Practice
• Time	• Educational	• Time Investment
• Finances	• Teaching	• Accessibility
• Retirement	• Organizational	• Patient Load
	• Non-Medical Activities	• Patient Mix
		• New Services
		• New Partner

Finances _____ In one of our recent marketing seminars, we asked doctors if their economic goals were part of their practice planning. Almost all agreed that economic goals were important, but only a few had taken the concept past the simple desire to maintain income growth. One was a colleague who was looking ahead. She had enough business now, she said, but she'd soon have two boys in college "and that's when I'll need marketing help."

If your competitive environment has cut into your practice load, your immediate financial goal might be more patients, right away. But if you're satisfied with your current income, you might use marketing strategies to ensure progressive growth.

In identifying your personal and financial goals, it's wise to discuss them with your financial adviser, family members, partners, and colleagues. What they tell you may alter your thinking.

Here are five important personal questions to ask yourself before beginning your marketing plan:

1. What do I want from the practice of medicine?
2. What are my immediate and long-range practice goals in terms of personal involvements?
3. How much time do I need, now and future, for my family?
4. What are my economic needs today? What will they be in five years? Ten years? In retirement?
5. What are the demands that these economic goals will place on my practice?

PROFESSIONAL GOALS _____ One physician showed good insight into a potential marketing plan in noting his desire to do a lot of organizational work with his specialty society. He felt it would help bring in new patients and ease his concern about losing patients to competing forces. Further discussion, however, revealed that his medical society work would take a good deal of time away from his practice. So his actual problem wasn't so much patient generation as it was patient retention, with maximum utilization of his time. After a thorough evaluation, we strongly recommended that he concentrate on marketing techniques to streamline his practice, and to delegate more responsibility.

For some idea of the many important decisions that may contribute to a similar understanding of your professional goals, ask yourself:

1. Am I satisfied with my current level of expertise?
2. Do I want to spend all my professional time practicing medicine exclusively?

3. Are there aspects of medicine, other than direct patient care, that are, or will be, important to me?
4. How much time do I want to spend teaching or in continuing education?
5. How will these professional goals affect overall practice plans?
6. What nonmedical activities would enhance my professional growth?

PRACTICE GOALS

Many physicians seem to know exactly how they want their practices to develop, but few are able to say what they think should be done to achieve their aims.

Recently, a physician asked us for help in attracting patients to his new practice in the Northeast. Many potential patients were going to the older, established physician in the community. When we offered that new hours might draw new patients, the young doctor interrupted, "I want you to know that my office hours are, and always will be, nine to five. I close for lunch, and I won't open on Saturdays."

With those words he all but slammed the door on his marketing options. Further investigation revealed that the competing physician was attracting many new patients by doing precisely what our young friend said he'd never do. The older doctor was staying open later in the day to attract new workers who had recently moved into town when the major local industry went on a two-shift schedule. Though the younger physician's product was actually superior, the potential patients would never get to find out unless he made himself more accessible—which he eventually, reluctantly, did.

Another goal you must set is the number of patients to see each day. This doesn't mean how many you *can* see, if forced to, but how many you *want* to see. One physician told us she'd take as many patients as she could get. But after some thought, she set a more plausible goal of 20 to 30 patients per day. No matter what competition exists, and tempting though it may be to shoot for the moon, you have to maintain a realistic attitude toward your practice goals.

Many physicians want marketing help not just in building their practices, but in shaping them. One doctor may be concerned because his practice consists of mostly geriatric patients. Even though he enjoys this area of medicine, he may be seeking ways to attract more young people and widen his patient mix.

Another doctor may need marketing help when trying to decide whether to bring in another partner. The big question in this case: Is there enough current business, or enough prospects of future growth, to justify another physician? Any number of imponderables may determine the answer.

For example: A four-doctor, family-practice group in the South had all the work it could handle; the decision was to add another body. But just as the new man came on board, a rival three-doctor group opened down the street. In the face of that competition, it took three years and much good marketing technique for the five-member group to build its practice to sufficient strength.

So before making any decision, ask yourself:

1. How much time am I willing to spend practicing medicine?
2. How accessible am I willing to be to my patients?
3. How many patients am I willing to see per day?
4. Am I satisfied with my current patient mix?
5. Do I plan to expand my practice by adding new services and/or another physician?

Setting goals for a practice isn't always easy, especially when they involve personal needs. But it must be done if you want to build a workable marketing plan. (Appendix A is a "Physician Self-Assessment Survey" to help clarify your personal and professional goals.)

PRACTICE ASSESSMENT
When you've concluded your assessment of where you are, and where you want to be personally and professionally, you must begin to look critically at the vehicle that will take you there—your medical practice. Again, it isn't easy to analyze your life's work. We're impressed, of course, by doctors who take a great deal of personal pride in their offices and how they are run. They should. But this protectiveness can often interfere with an objective and accurate judgment of strengths and weaknesses. *(See Fig. 3-B)*

A consultant friend asked one such physician why he was seeking help with a marketing plan. The reply: "Because I'm losing a lot of my patients to the competition."

"Do you think any are leaving because of your practice?"

"Absolutely not!" he snorted. "I've worked for 15 years to build this practice, and I can tell you that when patients leave it has nothing to do with anything that's wrong with my practice."

"Then why are they leaving?"

After a long hesitation, the physician quietly responded, "I don't know."

Ultimately, he had to face it: There *were* some things wrong with his practice, but nothing that couldn't be corrected by using the right marketing principles. We sympathize with such doctors. If you've devoted your whole professional life to perfecting your practice, it's

Figure 3-B
ASSESSING YOUR PRACTICE

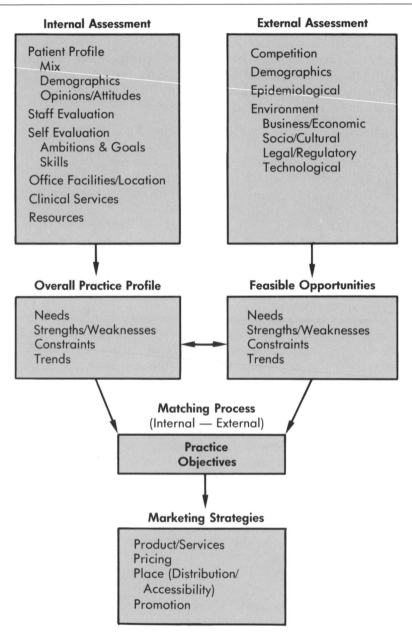

Internal Assessment

Patient Profile
   Mix
   Demographics
   Opinions/Attitudes
Staff Evaluation
Self Evaluation
   Ambitions & Goals
   Skills
Office Facilities/Location
Clinical Services
Resources

External Assessment

Competition
Demographics
Epidemiological
Environment
   Business/Economic
   Socio/Cultural
   Legal/Regulatory
   Technological

Overall Practice Profile

Needs
Strengths/Weaknesses
Constraints
Trends

Feasible Opportunities

Needs
Strengths/Weaknesses
Constraints
Trends

Matching Process
(Internal — External)

**Practice
Objectives**

Marketing Strategies

Product/Services
Pricing
Place (Distribution/
   Accessibility)
Promotion

Courtesy of Peter M. Sanchez, PhD, Villanova University.

hard to admit that your creation may be imperfect. As a result, most physicians will base their assessment on a hunch, a guess, a personal bias—anything but the hard look that might disclose an intrinsic flaw in their "baby."

To get you started in thinking about it, we'll first tackle the issue of competition. Then we'll look at demographic and economic considerations, and examine the major elements in your practice that may affect a marketing effort.

Your Competitors

The competitive environment varies from practice to practice, and from location to location. In many parts of the country, the major threat is the freestanding, primary-care center. In other places, it might be the physician surplus, an HMO, or even the local hospital. No matter where the threat is coming from, you have to be able to identify the competition. Here's a list of questions to help you do it:

1. Have you had an unusual number of recent requests for the transfer of records?
2. Where have you been sending those records?
3. Have you noticed announcements of new practices opening in your neighborhood?
4. Have new members been added to the hospital staff or the medical society? Are they potential competitors?
5. Have specialists and subspecialists been broadening their practices to treat a greater variety of patient situations?
6. Have any new primary-care or emergency centers opened?
7. Has local industry initiated, or been talking about, sending employees to a prepaid health facility?

A thorough look at those and related questions will generally show who your competitors are. And don't forget to ask your office staff those same questions, because they often become well aware of the trends before you do.

Once you've identified your competitors, get to know about them, and determine their strengths, weaknesses, and marketing activities. With that data you can plan what marketing weapons you need to combat them.

New Services. Of course, it would be myopic to think your only competition comes from fellow physicians. There are three categories of *other* competitors. First, there are those who try to satisfy by offering a new and different service based on the very general principle that the public is primarily interested in "feeling good." So psychic heal-ers, wellness centers, and other nonmedical and even nonphysical services are, in many ways, competing effectively by trying to make people "feel better" without the use of traditional medical care.

Nonphysician Specialists. The second type of competition comes from those who believe a particular service can be provided by a wide range of nonphysician "specialists." For example: The exercise craze has spawned a large number of sports complexes and smaller facilities. They instruct people on how to get and stay healthy through exercise. This advice, once dispensed primarily by physicians, can now be found in almost any shopping center, mall, or storefront health club. Many feel the alternative providers have been spawned largely by the physicians' lack of interest in providing these services.

The same applies to the field of nutrition. Nonmedical specialists now have private practices to attract people who don't get, or don't want to get, nutritional advice from a doctor. Health food stores are another form of this competition, providing both the products and the advice.

Alternative Care. The third type of competition comes from within the medical world from organizations that can provide the same services physicians do, but in different settings. Hospitals, for example, now deliver outpatient care through primary-care centers and surgical-outpatient clinics. They're particularly effective because they're usually large enough to have the dollars and work force to compete.

Each type of alternative care offers a different style of competition that you have to understand before you can use counter-marketing tactics. The first type of competitor, for example, is using different services to satisfy patient needs that you should be satisfying. Your marketing strategy would be to find ways to convince the public that you, the doctor, can make them feel better than, say, a wellness specialist can.

Sadly, in many cases, the doctor simply defaults to the competitors by appearing not to be concerned with a patient's need to feel better apart from the treatment of a specific medical problem. We forget that before World War II, making patients "feel better" about their illness was one of the doctor's major talents.

The advent of our miracle drugs and intricate surgical procedures has tended to make many of us rely too much on the science of medicine, and too little on the art of healing in all its more intangible forms. The famous painting of the concerned doctor sitting at the side of what is obviously a grievously ill patient was not just an artist's fancy. It was not unusual for doctors to do just that, for hours, in an attempt to give the patient some feeling of strength and hope.

We're not suggesting that you spend all your already precious time that way. But you must become concerned with the patient's desire for "wellness," and you must develop ways to satisfy that need. If you don't, your patients will go wherever they can get the understanding that you may have failed to give them—and they'll tell their friends.

Another reason why the sympathetic competitor has thrived is because doctors have failed to provide some of the special services patients need. Look at obesity: For years, many physicians have been treating overweight patients by handing them a diet and expecting them to follow it without motivation or direction. Patients who needed more than that—and virtually all do—had to wait until other formats were developed to provide this service. And developed they were, and with a vengeance. Independent dietitians, nutritionists, exercise specialists, and others have flourished by catering to the need to reduce weight.

Physicians should be competing for those patients by structuring their practices to incorporate such services or, at the very least, have one of the competitors affiliated with their practice.

The third type of competition, coming from the traditional providers—hospitals—is the most difficult to counter because in most cases they provide services similar to those you provide, and in settings acceptable to patients.

Health Plans. A major new competitor may also become an ally—the health plan. Spurred by the growing cost of medical care, such plans cut deals with employer groups and providers—both physicians and hospitals. Whatever the framework—HMO, IPA, or PPO—the health plans are forcing increasing numbers of physicians to either join, or do battle with them. The issue boils down to weighing the advantages of trading a certain amount of practice independence for entry to a new source of patients.

Demographic Assessment
Early in the evaluation of your practice environment, you must also look at your demographics. This involves taking a mini-census of where your patients live, and how they're divided according to such characteristics as age, sex, and illness. How can this help you? Well, here are a few examples:

A pediatrician expressed concern that his practice seemed to be drying up. How could we help him find out if it was? We started by spending several hours going through his assessment of practice goals, and we were impressed that he seemed to have his objectives in focus. Then we asked if he had ever looked at his community and tried to identify population trends and changes.

He laughed, "Hey, I'm a doctor, not a census taker."

But after we explained its importance, he agreed to spend one Saturday afternoon with us conducting a demographic survey.

Here's what we found: First, his practice was located in an older part of the county. Then a quick look at the records at the county seat clearly showed that the population was thrusting out on the other side of the city.

"What's the meaning of this for me?" he asked. "When I started this practice 15 ago there were more than enough patients. Just because the other side of town is growing, doesn't mean my area is shrinking, does it?"

We pointed out that it wasn't the total population that was moving to the other side of town, but the *younger* families.

"Oh, right, and the younger families are where I find my patients."

"That's it. So your practice is probably 'drying up' because your patients are getting older and your potential patient growth area is too far from your office."

"I just remembered," he groaned, "that's where the new young pediatrician just located. Smart kid."

Demographic fact-finding isn't always that simple. But it's always informative. Another physician, in the Midwest, was concerned about not seeing many older patients. He had a particular interest in geriatrics and wanted to attract more seniors into his practice. His demographic survey quickly revealed that more than 75 percent of his patients lived in the southern and southwestern parts of the county, but that the major retirement communities, retirement homes, and nursing homes were in the eastern section.

Since the major sources of referral for new patients are current patients, it was obvious that his current clientele were not living in an area where other older people were moving in. Consequently, they had few referrals to offer the doctor. No wonder he wasn't attracting new business.

With this demographic information, however, he focused his marketing efforts in the heavily geriatric eastern section, and within six months his over-60 patient population jumped by 25 percent.

Here are some more things to look for in your demographic survey:

Population Trends. You'll want to look at the trends in population growth, identify the direction in which the population is moving, and determine where the largest number of new families live. You'll also want the location of the newest subdivisions and where new construction permits have been granted. It's then a matter of selecting the areas in which you wish to concentrate.

Figure 3-C
ASSESSING YOUR LOCATION

The Community	Your Practice
• Population	• Accessibility
• Age Distribution	• Patient Convenience
• Economy	• Personal Convenience
	• Proximate Competition

Age Distribution. Not only can you pinpoint the age distribution of residents in specific areas, you can use these data to focus on patients with a particular disease. Arthritis and heart problems, for example, will be found primarily among the older populations.

Economic Trends. Occasionally, the growth of a practice may be slowed because the economy of the area has declined. Unemployment may be up because of business closings or factory layoffs. If you find such trends in your area, your practice will probably reflect the changes. Inquire about the chances for future growth, and where and when it might come. A slowing economy limits your plans for immediate growth, and could signal long-range problems you should prepare to face. But it needn't be a cause for alarm.

Think Before You Move. Practice location in an area of declining population or economic deterioration doesn't automatically suggest that you should move. Too many doctors jump the gun and head for new locations when those conditions appear. They often leave behind potentially lucrative practice areas, if only they had taken the trouble to "mine" them with the right marketing procedures. So, if you feel you're in this position, look before you leap: Consider your demographic and economic assessments in comparison with your competition before making a move. *(See Fig. 3-C)*

Following is a list of the major areas to include in a survey of factors outside your office that may affect your practice, and the places you can get the information you need:

1. Population growth or decline: Office of planning and development, office of building permits, board of education (to check on the opening or the closing of schools).
2. Economic growth or decline: Chamber of commerce, better business bureau, local bank officials (for local unemployment

figures, number of housing starts, defaults on loans and mort-
gages, etc.).
3. Technological growth: Chamber of commerce and governmental agencies dealing with new industrial growth. In larger metropolitan areas, banks, newspapers, and bureaus of
business and economic research in colleges and universities
may provide additional sources of information.

Appendix B is a detailed demographic survey and analysis you can
adjust to your particular needs. Collecting the needed data may seem
to be a monumental task, but it can usually be accomplished by your
office staff, or you may want to hire a business major at a local college
or university to assist you. When the survey is completed, take a long
look at the environment in which your practice is located and ask
yourself these questions:

1. Is my practice in the center of the population growth areas?
2. Is the population shifting away from my location?
3. Is the economy of my area declining? If yes, are there plans to
reverse it?

Although you can't control the demographic or economic factors, the
data you gather will help you develop marketing strategies to blunt
the bad effects they can have on your practice.

Internal Assessment
Once your external demographic and
economic survey is completed, your self-assessment must continue
with an examination of the strengths and weaknesses of your internal
environment—that is, what goes on in your office.

Your Physical Plant. How your office appears is one of the top criteria
your patients use in judging your services. All physicians want to be
thought of as providing quality service. The irony is that patients actually *can't* judge your quality accurately. Instead, they use what
marketing experts call "surrogate perceptions."

Patients get strong impressions from your office environment. Why
not? What other yardsticks do they have to measure you by? They're
not medical experts, so they have no way of judging your technical
expertise. All that's left to them is your manner and appearance. And
those start with your reception area, office, examining rooms, and
overall outward appearances.

On a recent visit at a friend's office, we were shocked by the appearance of the reception area. (Incidentally, it's always "the reception
area," never "the waiting room." Who needs to be reminded that patients have to wait?) It was bleakly decorated, badly furnished, and

poorly lit. Patients were obviously ill at ease in uncomfortable chairs. The overall effect was that of an aging bus station.

We knew this doctor well and we were surprised that a man of his ability would practice in such an unappealing atmosphere. We tactfully mentioned the effect his reception area had upon us.

His reply was surprising: "I know it's atrocious, but it would cost a fortune to fix it up. Besides, my patients come to see me, not my office.

"Anyway," he continued, as if the subject was unimportant, "what I need is some help. I've been in this practice 10 years, and I can't figure out why it's going downhill."

We didn't pursue the obvious right away, but after we'd assessed his practice, we had to make him see that his physical plant was in need of a face-lift. "Patients may come to see you, as you say," we told him, "but no matter how well you may treat them medically, a good number are going to be turned off and go away for good, just because of the gloom and discomfort of waiting in your reception area and examining rooms.

"Look at it this way: If you can immediately tell patients what's wrong with them, and start them on a prompt course of treatment that will bring quick results, they may not worry about how your plant looks. But what about the delayed diagnoses, the trial and error period when you may have to experiment with various treatments? Knowing they have to come here, maybe every week, to wait in this room could result in driving them away."

He put up no further argument. His office environment wasn't his only problem, of course. But it was a key to the way his patients regarded him and his abilities: A bus station office might very well harbor a bus station doctor.

In assessing the appeal of your office, ask yourself:

1. Is my reception area clean?
2. Is it physically appealing?
3. Is it comfortable? Will older patients and those with joint or muscular problems find it difficult to get in and out of my chairs?
4. Are there enough places to sit, or am I wedging my patients in like cattle?
5. Are my office colors bright and cheerful?
6. Are the examining rooms comfortable? Warm enough? Cool enough? Drafty? Cheerful? Have I put up a poem, a picture, something upbeat for them to look at, and something to read while waiting?
7. If I visited this office, would I see the overall operation as having quality?

That doesn't mean you have to spend a lot of money on expensive interior decorating. But you should provide a pleasing and comfortable environment if you want to give your patients the impression that you're a quality doctor who cares about their feelings and is considerate when it comes to their comfort.

Your Medical Staff. You can have a beautiful office, and you can be the finest doctor in the state delivering the best of medical care. But if your patients see your staff as unfriendly, or even openly hostile, you could find all your efforts undermined.

For example: We dealt with a five-member practice in the East that was having problems. A self-assessment revealed that four of the partners were unhappy with the office manager, feeling she was unsympathetic to patients' needs. The fifth member, the managing partner, was unaware of his colleagues' unhappiness, and was astounded to find that the office manager had indeed been driving people away by refusing to work with unpaid accounts.

Many physicians are stunned to find how much patient dissatisfaction can be created by staff members who refuse to meet patients' most simple and reasonable needs.

One doctor, whose practice relied on referrals, was surprised to learn that his secretary was refusing to take patients referred by another physician. Confronted, she told how that referring physician had once called the office demanding certain appointment times for his patients, and since then she'd been "getting even" by turning away his referrals. In other cases, staff members have been known to refuse such simple courtesies as telling patients about their blood pressure readings.

The success or failure of a practice depends very largely on staff attitudes. So one of your basic moves should be to assess their contributions. Ask these questions about them:

1. Does my receptionist or secretary really meet the needs of my patients? What have I heard her do and say? What comments about her have I heard?
2. Do patients complain that they can't get appointments when they need them?
3. Are there complaints about not receiving help with insurance forms or with straightening out overdue accounts?
4. Is my nursing staff responding to the needs of my patients?
5. Do I feel that the staff, in general, is friendly and courteous to patients?
6. If I were a patient, how would I rate the staff?

7. Does the staff understand the services I provide, and my goals for the future?
8. Are they able to communicate to patients an understanding of my services? Do patients leave the office thinking they have to go elsewhere for a service they don't know I provide?

Physicians are often unable to judge their staff members without personal bias. Yet the success of your marketing efforts depends on an accurate assessment. How accurate you are will be revealed later, when you complete your patient survey.

Your Patient Mix. Many physicians never evaluate their patient load except in terms of numbers. And while numbers are important, other factors must also be considered. For example: What types of patients do you see? Are the majority over 55? If yes, then you definitely have a problem. Not many primary-care practices can survive for long on mostly older patients, except in very heavy retirement areas. Referral practices, too, must consider whether they are seeing the types of patients they really need in order to realize their practice goals.

Your Services. This is the cornerstone of your practice. You must be certain you're providing services that match your practice goals and your patients' needs. At the same time, you must be fully aware of how patients regard your services. Unfortunately, surveys of the internal environments rarely include the physicians' own understandings of what they provide. At the very least, you should be able to list all of your services and to decide whether you're meeting all the varied needs of your patient mix.

When you conduct an internal assessment of your patient mix and the services you provide, ask these questions:

1. What types of patients make up my practice?
2. Am I satisfied with the variety of patients I see?
3. Does my patient mix meet both my short- and long-term practice goals?
4. What attracts my current patients to my practice?
5. Why might potential patients choose another practice?
6. What are the main services I provide?
7. Are my patients aware of all my services?
8. Are there any services I don't now offer, that I could offer?
9. Given the opportunity, how would I go about changing the services I provide?

Appendix C provides a more detailed practice survey questionnaire. Complete it so you can pinpoint your strengths and weaknesses.

Summary —————————————— To improve your practice position in
the medical marketplace, you must know your current strengths and
weaknesses, and where you stand in your competitive environment. A
thorough self-assessment is essential in evaluating potential changes,
and in expanding your present assets. Even if you already occupy a
good position, an assessment can show you how to strengthen it by
matching your perceptions with those of your patients. You should be
aware of the relationship between the external and internal assessments of your practice and the development of your ultimate marketing strategies.

CHAPTER 4

Market research can tell you what's wrong

Before you can begin to think about marketing strategies, you have to determine how your customers—your patients—view your practice, why they perceive it that way, and how they would like to see it change.

You can try to get this information in two ways—by intuitive estimates or by marketing research. In some situations, intuitive estimates work well. But since they're often based on guesswork, hunches, or unconscious bias, the conclusions frequently aren't what patients had in mind at all. You may be very concerned about the health of your patients, but that's not the same as being oriented to their *needs,* or what's more important, what they *think* their needs are. Their real or fancied needs may often involve matters peripheral to their general health.

To understand your patients it's necessary to share—or at least empathize with—their concerns and opinions. And the greater the social distance between you and them, the less your intuitive powers will be able to pick up on what's in their hearts and minds. All of which leaves you with marketing research as your best instrument.

The technical definition of marketing research is "the systematic gathering, recording, and analyzing of data pertaining both to the marketing of a service and to the consumers of that service." A good, stuffy, academic definition. Let's put it in plain English: You must learn what you're selling, and what your patients want to buy.

WHAT IS MARKET RESEARCH FOR YOU?

What you want are new facts and insights—not verifications of your own biases. As a physician you've been trained to gather facts in exacting detail about disease and treatments. You've done this sort of thing many times before, but in scientific contexts. So the inherent logic in the marketing-research process should be right up your alley.

This chapter will show you how to nail down your best method of organizing the search for facts. We'll cover the writing of clear and definite objectives, how your facts can be gathered completely and without prejudice, and how to piece them together in an understandable manner. *(See Figs. 4-A, 4-B)*

Organize the Search

At first glance, it may seem that you're looking for any information to help you evaluate your practice. That could be exhausting and wasteful. Instead, you must organize your research so that it covers the specific areas that apply to your unique situation.

Although patients are the focus of most physician marketing research, you can use this same research process in generating information on any outside group affecting your practice, such as referring physicians, employers, insurance companies, and competitors.

To understand most of the *external* groups, you'll need some general research material. You'll often find this published in applied medical

Figure 4-A
STEPS IN MARKETING RESEARCH

1. Determine Your Objectives
2. Conduct an Informal Investigation
3. Determine Needed Information
4. Prepare the Survey Forms
5. Decide on Method of Gathering Data
6. Pretest the Survey
7. Collect the Data
8. Analyze and Interpret the Results

Figure 4-B
EXTERNAL IMPACTORS ON YOUR PRACTICE

- Patients
- Employers
- Insurance Companies
- Competitors
- Others

and business periodicals. Regular reading of a variety of these publications, such as *American Medical News* and *Business Week,* is vital to keeping informed on the changing medical marketplace. Some of the trends you read about may help you form ideas for your own patient survey.

Do It Yourself _____ Let's turn back to the topic of your own surveys. It's essential that you collect data in all areas that directly or indirectly affect your patients. Organization is critical, so if you solicit opinions from patients in only a few areas, and in an ill-structured fashion, you'll end up with a distorted picture.

We'll provide a suggested outline for your survey. While other areas may be important for your specific practice, the outline will set the framework for your overall analysis. To begin, you need to find out how your patients feel about your:

Specialty	Competitors	Offices
Nurses	Fees	Partners
Receptionists	Availability	Ancillary Services

You must also find out your patients' needs and wants in these areas:

Scheduling appointments	Time spent with you
Information from you	Services from you

Chapter 5 has a more detailed discussion of each of those areas, and Appendix D is a complete and tabulated patient survey.

Draft the Questions _____ If you expect unbiased answers, be careful how you phrase your questions. The way a question is asked can predetermine the answer.

Take, for example, a question designed to gather information on your after-hours care. Let's say you're asking patients about their experience with having their phone calls returned. Your question could be phrased this way:

Figure 4-C
RESEARCH QUESTIONS

- Factual
- Opinion and Attitude
- Informational
- Self-Perception

"Has the doctor ever failed to return your call?" Most patients would automatically answer No. That would make you feel good, but the question really didn't offer patients a way to give you an evaluation of the quality of your service.

You'll get much more meaningful information if you ask the question in a way that allows patients to express their feelings about your effectiveness: "Does the doctor return your calls promptly?"

Be careful not to lead your respondents in one direction or another. Leave them free to give their uninfluenced opinions.

Put your queries in logical order, grouped according to subject areas. Don't ask, for example, "How many children do you have? What are their ages? Sex?" and then, "Are you married, single, or widowed?" It's not a blunder, but the questions are out of the normal sequence and obviously should be reversed. Don't jar patients any more than necessary. And, finally, keep your questions simple and easy to understand, and to answer.

Who Are Your Patients? There are four types of survey questions. First, there are those that seek the *facts*, the simple personal and demographic details: name, age, address, marital status, children, occupation, education, and income. That seems simple enough, but there are traps. The name, for example. How important is it for you to know exactly who answered each particular questionnaire? Some people might not answer as honestly if they give their names, as they would if they remained anonymous. *(See Fig. 4-C)*

They may be afraid to criticize your practice for fear of angering you. You probably need not fear losing such patients; they're probably too conservative to switch doctors except under the direst pressures. But if they have hidden doubts, fears, or criticisms of your practice, the chances of their sending you referrals are remote. So if the name of the respondent isn't a critical factor, skip it.

Marital status, however, *is* vital information. Physicians may not always be aware of how many of their patients are married, single, or single parents. The last category is a sensitive one. Single parents are usually working parents, and are almost totally absorbed in making ends meet and taking care of their children. Finding time to see a doctor may require major planning.

The number of children in a family is equally important. Many primary care physicians are amazed to find that a large percentage of their patients have children who are being cared for by other doctors. You'll also want to know if there are other family members who could be receiving their health care from you, but who don't. Not many grandparents, maiden aunts, or bachelor uncles are living in nuclear families these days. But there are some. Your patients may be taking their elderly mothers and fathers elsewhere because they're unaware that you might welcome treating older people.

Demographics. In Chapter 3 we indicated the importance of a demographic survey to assess your practice and to find where your patients are concentrated. You can do this easily by asking for home addresses and zip codes. By plotting these on a map of your community, you can quickly identify where your patients are coming from, and spot the areas from which you may not be drawing your fair share. You've then identified one of your problems, and can make plans to remedy the trouble.

Schedules. Many of your patients have jobs that occupy them more than eight hours a day and that send them on frequent trips. Their time is limited. Also, the trend is for both husband and wife to work. So, if both partners are at their jobs all day, it obviously makes access to health care more difficult. Think of your own situation. If you have to see your doctor, how easy is it for you to break out of your workday to do it? Or how about seeing your accountant, or attorney, or any one of a half-dozen professionals you might have to consult?

You appreciate being able to see them after hours, before starting your day, or on weekends, right? Well, now you're empathizing with your working patients. Given those circumstances, it's not hard to see one big reason for the popularity of convenience clinics.

Survey Sample. Here's a sample of the FACT questions that are important for a thorough patient survey:

Name (optional)	Marital Status
Spouse & Children	Ages
Education	Occupation(s)
Home Address	Phone
Work Address	Phone

Other family members living with you
Other sources of health care you use
Best times for appointments

What Do They Think of You? The second type of question, and probably the most useful, concerns *opinions* and *attitudes*—what respondents think of certain aspects of your practice. A major criticism of most surveys and polls is that they often reflect respondents' subjective responses, not the facts. But those subjective responses are *exactly* what you're after, because their opinions determine whether patients will stay with you, and whether you can attract new ones.

How Much Do They Know? The third type—the *informational* question—is used to gauge the respondent's knowledge of specific subject matter, primarily, the nature of your specialty and services. At least one of your questions should be aimed at finding out how much your patients know about the scope of your work. Many haven't the faintest notion of what specific health care you provide. Some, it's true, will come to you, faithfully, to seek the diagnosis and cure of everything from a hangnail to cancer. But too many may be thinking you have a very limited range and be going to specialists for services you can provide.

How Good Is Their Judgment? The fourth type of survey question involves *self-perception*. Here, respondents are asked to evaluate certain entities or actions, such as alternative delivery systems. Construct questions that will elicit answers to what conditions in your practice might be driving patients to choose other health-care sources. The reasons may have nothing to do with your quality of service, but you must find out. And you have to get specific. For example:

1. Do you, or would you, consider utilizing other facilities to receive part of your health care?
2. If you have used other facilities, what were they, and what was your reason for doing so?
3. Are there specific problems that you find in our practice that would lead you to consider going elsewhere for your health needs?

Construct the Questions

As a rule of thumb, make your questions brief, easy to understand, and easy to answer. They should be worded to be understood by a patient with no more than an 8th-grade education. That isn't meant to insult your patients. Most people—even "brilliant doctors"—respond best to questions at an 8th-grade level of comprehension. If you walked into your lawyer's office and were handed a questionnaire designed to find out how you viewed the law firm's services, wouldn't you appreciate having the questions phrased simply? Or would you prefer to engage in an intellectual wrestling match with overblown language? Worse yet, how would you like your attorney to phrase his questionnaire in legalese? The answer is obvious. You appreciate good, simple English. So does everyone else.

Because physicians may have a tendency to get wordy, or technical in their language, it's a good idea to have your most literate staff member put your questionnaire in final form, or at least edit what you've written.

Divide your questionnaire with headings that reflect your organizational outline, and make your questions the "yes" or "no" type. Questions requiring written responses are less likely to be answered, and are more difficult to analyze. You may want to incorporate a few, particularly those that encourage respondents to outline what it is that displeases them.

Design the Research

When the questionnaire is complete, it's time to establish the methods for carrying out the survey. This is the point where physicians often balk, because they're hesitant about plunging into a time-consuming project they aren't sure is worth the effort. But if you understand the basic techniques, you can administer the survey quite efficiently with very little loss of your time. There are four basic ways to go about it (see Fig. 4-D):

Telephone. We're all familiar with marketing research carried out via the phone, because we've all been on the receiving end. The caller asks a series of questions and records the answers. It's efficient, inexpensive, and can be done after regular office hours. However, people are often suspicious of talking to someone they don't know and can't see. As a result, they may give less than honest opinions. Of course, that

Figure 4-D
SURVEY TECHNIQUES

Type	Advantages	Disadvantages
Telephone Behavior	Efficient Inexpensive	Less Reliable Time Restraints
Mail Questionnaire	Able to Sample Patient Convenience No Interviewer Bias	Expensive Time Consuming Less Response
Direct Interview	Direct Contact Better Explanation Flexible Higher Return	Interviewer Bias

won't be a serious problem when you're calling your longtime patients. The phone can be a barrier, though, to new patients who don't yet know you very well.

Mail. Mailing questionnaires has several advantages. They can be sent to a select sampling of patients, and you're not dependent on interview subjects coming to your office. Both you and your respondents have the luxury of dealing with the survey at times convenient to each of you. You can also cover a wide geographic area without leaving the office, and—quite important—the mailed questionnaire removes any interviewer bias in the way questions are asked. Using the mails can be quite expensive, however, because you should provide a stamped, self-addressed envelope to ensure a high response. Also keep in mind that a mail survey takes considerable time to complete, and that those who do respond may not constitute a representative sampling of your patient population.

Interview. This is the survey method often chosen by physicians. Since the personal interview involves direct contact, you can better explain the purpose and content of the questionnaire, person to person. It also elicits more information from the patient.

The great advantage of the personal interview is that your percentage of return is virtually guaranteed. Few people refuse to participate. Of course, there are limitations to this method, too—primarily the possibility for bias on the part of both the interviewer and the interview subject.

Self-Administration. The personal interview approach can be modified by having the patients fill out the questionnaire on their own, following a short briefing by a staff member. That decreases the possibility of bias, and also makes your staffers available, if needed, to help patients understand the questions.

Sampling

Two major criteria must be met before your survey can provide a complete assessment: The sampling must be adequate in size, and it must be representative. You can't draw marketing conclusions from only a small portion of your patients. Surveying your entire practice would be a tremendous task, so you must find a number that will reflect majority opinions.

That number depends on how many patients you have. If you're well established, a good cross section will be 15 to 20 percent. So if you have, say, 2,000 patients, you'll need 300 to 400 responses. For physicians not fully established, a good sampling will consist of responses equal to five times the daily average of patient visits. If you see 15 patients a day, for example, you'll need at least 75 responses.

Since not everyone will respond, you have to distribute more questionnaires than the number you need for a valid assessment. How many should you distribute? It depends on how you're conducting your survey.

If you're handing the questionnaire to patients in your office, expect about an 80 percent return. So if you need 300 responses, you'll probably have to hand out at least 375 questionnaires. If you're mailing them, expect only about a 50 percent return.

To meet the second criterion—a representative cross section of your patient population—you'll have to exercise some personal judgment, according to your type of practice. Specialists not dealing in primary care will see about the same patient mixture throughout the year. Surgeons, for example, will be seeing people who need surgery, often specific types of surgery.

But primary-care physicians see so many different segments of the population, and with seasonal variations, that deciding whom to survey, and when, can vary greatly from doctor to doctor. Do you survey in the pollen season when allergy sufferers are beating down your door? In mid-winter, when everyone is wheezing with pulmonary problems? Do you start your survey just as a mini-epidemic of gastrointestinal problems hits town and your office is full of people with stomach aches? So, when it comes to when to survey, you have to rely on your own good judgment. Now let's examine the three basic ways to choose whom you will interview.

Random Sampling. In this method, every member of your active practice has an equal chance of being included. You may decide, for example, to pick every 10th patient who visits you over a period of, say, one month. This technique gives very representative results, but it's costly in the time spent planning and administering it.

Stratified Sampling. In this method you survey the exact percentages that make up your patient mix. If your practice is 50 percent geriatrics, 25 percent pediatrics, and 25 percent internal medicine, you'd survey according to those percentages and categories. This is the most representative method, but as you can see, it's also extremely time consuming, and probably the most costly.

Convenience Sampling. It's convenient because you survey those who are most available. You give questionnaires to all patients who come into your office over a period of time. The period is determined by the number of surveys required to reach your sampling number. This

Figure 4-E
SAMPLING TECHNIQUES

Type	Advantages	Disadvantages
Random Sample	Representative	Costly
Stratified Sample	Most Representative	Most Costly Most Time Consuming
Convenience Sample	Convenient Less Expensive Simplest	Less Scientific

convenient method is the least scientific, but it's the simplest and the least expensive. In the long run, the data collected often reflect enough patient characteristics and attitudes to make assessments of problem areas possible. *(See Fig. 4-E)*

Administer the Survey _____ You've now planned the major portion of your marketing research. All that's left is deciding how to run the show. We're sorry to say that physicians are usually the worst members of the practice to handle this task. They don't have the time, and even if they do, they can be very intimidating to the interviewees. Patients are less likely to give honest responses to the doctor. They are generally more comfortable when a staff member handles the questionnaire, or when they complete the survey by themselves.

The ideal person to handle the survey is your receptionist or secretary. He or she should already have a friendly rapport with the majority of your patients, and should be able to explain the purpose of the questionnaire without influencing respondents. The ideal time to approach patients, questionnaires in hand, is when they check in for their appointments. The purpose of the survey should be explained, and the patient should be asked to start filling it out while waiting for the doctor.

Why Patients Respond. Several important points must be emphasized by the one who hands the patient a questionnaire. First, the purpose of the survey must be explained. Simply put, it's to help re-evaluate your practice so you can provide better and more efficient health care. Most of your patients will be pleased to take an active role and give their opinions. They'll want to participate in a decision-making process that directly affects them. It asks for their input, and makes them feel that they're helping to provide direction for you—as indeed they are.

Patient Instructions. Each patient should be given both oral and printed instructions on what is expected of them in filling out the questionnaire. Make the instructions simple and to the point. Test your questionnaire, including the instructions, by letting some average 14-year-olds read it (assuming it's possible to find average 14-year-olds). If they have problems with either the instructions or the questions, so will some of your patients.

Here's an instruction list that works well:

1. Please answer all the questions.
2. If you don't know the answer, or don't have an opinion, place a question mark (?) in the answer space.
3. Answer as many questions as you can before seeing the doctor; answer the rest after your visit is over.
4. Please return your questionnaire to the secretary before you leave the office today.
5. If you have any questions, please ask the secretary. And thank you for your help.

Focus Group. Another survey research vehicle is the "focus group." It consists of eight to 12 people, patients and nonpatients. Composition of the group will be determined by your knowledge of your patients and associates, and by picking as representative a gathering as possible. A focus group can give you some in-depth opinions about your practice, your competition, specific health-care needs, and any other areas of interest.

Encourage the group to be critical. Urge them to pick at you. This has some of the features of group therapy sessions, except the subject of the therapy is your whole practice. To be productive, a focus group session has to be open and candid; you absolutely must not dominate it. In fact, you are there only as an "ear," not a voice. It's a good idea to have such a session before you design your questionnaire. You'll be amazed at the insights you'll gain.

Summary

You're now ready to start your marketing research. The main objective is to provide you with self-help guidelines. You should now be able to conduct your own search for the information you need. We've explored the technical aspects and provided examples that can be incorporated immediately into any practice, regardless of specialty.

You may be asking yourself: If marketing research is so necessary, why hasn't it been used more by physicians? The answer lies in the inherent fear of most physicians that it is "statistic-ridden" and "mysterious." In fact, it's neither. The techniques are simple. A thorough marketing survey can be carried out in any practice, big or small. Marketing research is how we find out "where we are." From there, it's up to us to decide where we want to go, and how to get there.

In the next chapter we'll see more of the specifics of conducting a patient survey, and examples of how responses to selected questions have benefited some practices.

CHAPTER 5

Find out what your patients really want

The keystones of your practice are your patients' needs and wants. Are you tired of having us harp on that point? We do it because it's so important. Doctors easily understand the point, intellectually. The trouble is that many maintain a gut resistance to it. If you're one of them, note this well: Until you realize that your *patients*, not *you*, are at the center of your professional world, you'll have an impaired practice, crippled by your own attitude.

In Search of Excellence finds authors Thomas Peters and Robert Waterman exploring the reasons major American companies have been successful. They discovered "that to these companies, the customer—his/her needs and wants—comes first, ahead of technology, ahead of cost." Story after story confirms that successful companies are, indeed, "people oriented" and "customer driven."[1]

Three main ingredients are cited. First, the company maintains a continuous, high standard of quality. Second, it maintains constant reliability in its performance. Third, and probably most important, it commits itself to identifying and meeting its customers' needs.

To describe the profession of medicine as "just another business" will quickly alienate most physicians. As well it should, because medicine is not "just" a business. It's much, much more. But it *is* a business, too, and it has to incorporate many features from the business world if it's to continue to effectively perform it's highest functions: prevention, diagnosis, and treatment of injuries and disease. To do that, medicine must have a commitment to its customers, not only to good medical treatment, but to satisfying patients' desires.

Applying the word "customers" to your patients probably makes you uncomfortable. (Didn't you feel a twinge of annoyance when we used the term earlier in the book?) After all, customers buy hardware, food, washing machines, automobiles. So how dare we call "patients" by that name? The objection is pedantic. Of course patients are customers, and no pejorative is implied or intended. Customers, clients, consumers, patients—all are acceptable synonyms for the people who buy health-care products and services. Each of us, no matter what our profession, constantly alternates in the roles of salesperson and customer. We trade what we know or what we can do for what other people are willing to pay us, and we are willing to pay others for what they know or can do for us.

In most cases, physicians are acutely attuned to the immediate health needs of their patients. They aren't accustomed, however, to changing their practices to satisfy the broader and less easily defined needs and wants of both current and potential patients. But once they find a way to identify those needs and wants, they'll be in a good position, like other successful business people, to structure their services to please the customer.

TAKING A SURVEY
THAT WORKS
In Chapter 4 we discussed the technical aspects of a patient survey. Now we'll examine the major questions necessary to create a marketing plan. *(See Fig. 5-A)*

Your Specialties

Question: Do you know what our special services can do for you? What is unique about your specialty? How comprehensive is the care you offer? Wouldn't it be frustrating to find, after all the expense and time invested in your training and experience, that many of your patients don't have the haziest idea of what you can really do? If you find that to be the case, you must educate them. For example:

Figure 5-A
AREAS FOR A PATIENT SURVEY

- Familiarity With Specialty
- Physical Environment
- Office Personnel
- Nursing Staff
- Partners

- Time Spent With Patients
- Time Spent Waiting
- Physician Accessibility
- Services Provided
- Pricing

After a survey, a doctor in a highly competitive area was astounded to find that her patients were unaware of her range of services. As a family physician, she knew that her very strength was in the comprehensiveness of her practice. Yet more than 50 percent of her customers used a pediatrician for their children, because most didn't know she treated youngsters. So her strategy had to include a major effort to inform patients about the full scope of her work, and to spread the word to potential consumers.

The failure of patients to fully understand their doctors' medical capabilities isn't confined to primary care. An ophthalmologist we encountered was interested in expanding his practice to include the field of contact lenses. He had spent several years gaining expertise, and was now ready to market his new medical interest. But he knew he'd be in direct competition with nonmedical businesses offering similar services.

In order to compete, he first had to find out how his potential patients viewed his specialty in comparison with the services offered by optometrists and other eye-care practitioners. To his relief, the survey revealed that people saw ophthalmologists as *the* experts in eye care. That was the green light for him to expand into full contact-lens care. When he did, he found his competitors far less of a threat than he'd anticipated.

Office

Question: Do you find our office convenient, comfortable, pleasing?
We've already noted that patients place great emphasis on the physician's physical plant. Because they use their perceptions of your facilities to judge the quality of your services—simple-minded as that may appear—you must pay close attention to their assessment of your office in terms of its location, comfort, and convenience.

"Damn it!" you're probably thinking. "What's all this frou-frou have to do with the practice of medicine?" Well, nothing, really, from *your* point of view. It has a lot to do with your practice, though, if you look at it from your patients' viewpoint.

You know exactly what you can do for your patients. But be logical, Doctor. How can your patients tell your value? They have no training that enables them to judge your medical abilities. They must rely on exterior appearances, just as you do when you're buying a product or service about which you know very little.

The average person can learn more about what car to buy than he can about what doctor's services he needs. There are no guides to the right doctor equivalent to consumer reports on automobiles or washing machines. No one publishes a book saying, "We've checked out Dr. Jones as compared with Dr. Smith, and Dr. Jones is superior." Your patients probably came to you purely on the advice of a friend, relative, or another doctor. They know nothing about you except what they may read on the diplomas and certificates on your walls. And have you noticed how many patients are too timid even to do that in your presence? They're afraid of offending you by demonstrating a lack of trust.

In a sense, some patients are like children. They're innocent and hopeful. Some may even fear you. They're becoming less so, getting bolder. Yet many are still fairly timid. Some fear that you won't cure them; others fear what you might do if they displease you.

So, arriving at your office, trusting the judgment of the person who referred them, or the happy accident of finding your name in the Yellow Pages, what real basis do they have for assessing what kind of doctor you are? The same basis you would have in visiting a new lawyer or accountant—really nothing more than the location and appearance of the professional office.

So you must ask if your location is easily accessible to a majority of your patients. Is ample parking nearby? Is your office a pleasant place to sit? If it is difficult to reach, patients might opt for more convenient service elsewhere. At first they might use those alternate services only in emergencies; eventually some will turn to them permanently for their care.

A two-physician partnership had documented a drop in average daily patient visits from 25 to 20. A demographic survey revealed that two primary-care centers (urgi-centers) had opened 18 months earlier. Worse yet, they were positioned between our physicians' office and the major patient population center. A patient survey showed that 65 percent of the customers saw our doctors' location as inconvenient. The reason for the falloff in patients was obvious. The urgi-centers were getting the customers.

Your physical environment extends into the reception area. What do you think of yours? Is it comfortable and pleasing? Would *you* like to wait there for a half hour? Many physicians are shocked to find their clientele complaining, not about the medical care, but about the lack of comfort in their facility. One group's survey showed that many geriatric patients had considered leaving their practice simply because the chairs in the reception area were so low that they had difficulty getting in and out of them. Imagine letting such a small detail play havoc with a business.

When we asked one physician if he thought his office environment was important to his practice, he said with great firmness, "Absolutely not!" We then guided him through a patient survey and, guess what? More than half his patients felt that his office *was* uncomfortable and unattractive. He soon changed it.

Staff

Question: Do you find our staff courteous, understanding, and sympathetic? Many excellent doctors have had their good efforts nullified by a hostile receptionist. As happens far more often than you might think, office personnel—with all good intentions—try to protect the doctor, and in the process damage the practice. So special attention should be paid to your staff's handling of patients, and to patients' reactions to your staff.

Figure 5-B
HOW CUSTOMERS ARE LOST

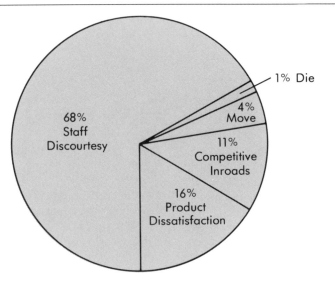

Why do customers leave one store for another with the same products or services? Most often, the reason is dissatisfaction—not with the products or services, but with the way the staff delivers them. The same applies to the delivery of physicians' services. *(See Fig. 5-B)*

So: Are your office helpers friendly and courteous? Are your phones answered promptly? Do your patients get the help they need with their money problems? Their insurance forms? Are your business policies adequately explained and carried out by your staff? If any answer is No, you've got a marketing problem that has to be fixed.

Nurses

Question: *Do you find our nurses courteous, understanding, and sympathetic?* While you may demonstrate a lot of empathy for your patients' problems, a rude or careless nurse can destroy that very quickly. Your nurses are a primary source of information for the patient. If they're not providing the needed information, they're turning off the customers.

One physician was concerned because a favorite patient asked that her records be forwarded to another doctor. He debated a long time, then decided to ask her, directly, if she was dissatisfied with him. She quickly reassured him that his medical care wasn't in question. She admitted, however, that she became very upset when she overheard a nurse laughing about her weight problem. She quite naturally interpreted the nurse's attitude as rude, uncaring, and indicative of the attitude of the entire practice. Despite anything the doctor could say, the patient left for good.

Partners

Question: *Do you feel that all the doctors in this practice care about you?* When you deal with patient opinions of your practice, you must include their assessment of your partners. Do they feel your colleagues take good care of them when you're unavailable? Or do they go elsewhere for care when you're not there?

We encountered a group of five internists who'd been together for several years. When asked about their professional relationships, the unanimous reply was, "Ideal." But several respondents to the patient survey reported having had difficulty reaching one of the partners when he was on call. That surprised the rest of the group, so they asked about it at the next office meeting. The accused doctor became unexpectedly angry and announced, "Look, I'm tired of getting called at all hours of the night for no good reason."

His attitude so surprised his associates that one of them called the man's wife and asked if everything was all right at home. She seemed to welcome the call and confessed that things were not all right. There were problems, but her husband wouldn't talk to anyone. Fortunately, the doctor who was closest to the couple was able to help the troubled physician work out some family problems, and his revealed deficiencies were dramatically reduced.

That incident demonstrates how the relationships between your partners and your patients (and your relationships with their patients) can have a strong influence on how customers perceive the entire practice.

A more common problem surfaced during a marketing consultation with an Oklahoma pediatric group. The survey revealed that 65 percent of their patients felt the other physicians in the group were not as concerned with their health care as was their own doctor. When this was brought up at a meeting, it stirred considerable discussion. The level of treatment rose markedly after that.

Time Spent With Patients

Question: Do the doctors spend enough time with you? Patients are remarkably sensitive to the time doctors spend with them. It's the one concern that's expressed over and over in surveys. They can't help comparing the time the doctor spends with them and the time they spend in the reception area. When they feel they're not getting their fair share of the doctor's attention, they may go to alternative providers. But note: What they're really asking for isn't *more* time, but *rapport* during the time together. They're asking for better *attention*.

We're all very poor judges of time. If patients see you as kind and understanding, 10 minutes may be enough to please them. If you're brusque and formal, no amount of time will satisfy them. Here's a case in point:

An internist's survey showed that her patients deplored the shortness of their meetings with her. She protested, "But I spend almost 20 minutes with each one." (Women doctors generally *do* tend to spend more time with each patient than do their male colleagues.)

We responded by asking her not to pay so much attention to the number of minutes, but to concentrate on spending "quality" time. "Make sure," we told her, "that you adequately explain their illness, the drugs required, and the possible course of the disease in a friendly, easy, unhurried fashion. That's what patients want. And make sure you find out whatever else may be troubling them. Further, when you're talking with them, never stand over them or sit on the examining table. Sit on their level and look them in the eyes."

The internist made a concerted effort to comply. When she repeated the survey six months later, only a few patients complained about the time spent with her. So the question not only revealed a marketing problem, it helped her give higher-quality care, and become a better doctor in the bargain.

In sum, it's important that you develop good communication skills, and be sure to:

1. Explain the illness thoroughly.
2. Discuss the tests you order.
3. Explain the reasons for the drugs you prescribe, what they can do, their side effects (if any), and why the patient's compliance is necessary.
4. Explain the possible course of the illness.

Time Patients Spend Waiting

Question: Do you have to wait too long to see the doctor? The 1980s may be remembered as the decade of "time." Major trends in business are being dictated by the consumers' preoccupation with the time they spend waiting for various services—medical care included. Many believe the major reason emergency rooms and convenience clinics have thrived is that people will no longer tolerate waiting patiently for medical care. If your patients think your practice doesn't value their time, they'll often find one that will.

A friend recently asked about a new doctor in town, indicating he would like an appointment. We told him the question was startling because he'd been going to the same doctor for more than a decade.

"Yeah, I know," he replied, "but he's gotten so busy it takes a week before you can see him. And when you get there you spend half a day waiting. Who can afford that? If he's got all the patients he can handle, he won't miss me."

The doctor doesn't have a marketing problem—yet. But he may be building up to one. When longtime patients begin moving on, trouble is brewing. So pay close attention to see if your survey reveals this sort of mutiny. If it does, do something to smooth out your appointment system. Consider lengthening your workday and/or devising better scheduling techniques to accommodate patients more rapidly.

Accessibility

Question: Can you reach the doctor when you need to? Patients want to feel they can reach you anytime they feel the need. When they lose that perception, it's often enough to make them switch doctors. That can quickly result in significant loss of patients. Here's what happened to an unsuspecting physician in the Southwest:

When he first began getting reports from an emergency center about visits his patients were making after his office hours, he wasn't at all alarmed. In fact, he welcomed the relief because he was feeling overworked. But he eventually found out that many of those patients were going to the emergency center *during* his office hours. A survey revealed that he was losing them simply because they couldn't reach him through his answering service. When he changed to another service, the problem vanished.

Remember, any time your phone is being covered by an answering service or another physician, the person on the phone is an extension of your practice—and a potential source of marketing problems. Perhaps the covering doctor isn't in the same type of practice, or doesn't share the same philosophy of care. Maybe he or she isn't interested in providing as high a quality of care, or will cover only well enough to get through the night. In any case, the lack of concern will be noticed by your patients, and is likely to cause you a number of major marketing headaches.

Remember, though, that while patients need to be educated about when to call after hours, they still must feel that help will be there whenever they need it.

They're also concerned about your accessibility during the day. Nationwide, physicians are reporting an increase in the number of phone calls during office hours. The consensus is that patients are trying to handle problems on the phone and save themselves the trouble—and the cost—of an office visit. When their calls aren't answered, they interpret it as your lack of interest.

Correcting that perception requires a great deal of patient education, and the close cooperation of your staff. No doctor can return every call immediately, but a system can be worked out that will satisfy both the physician's and the patient's needs. Train your staff to handle such calls, and organize a system to expedite return calls. Here are some good procedures to follow:

■ Have a set time, or times, each day for answering calls. A half hour first thing in the morning, a half hour at lunch, and a final half hour at the end of the day—that may well satisfy the callers without disrupting your office schedule.
■ Have your staff tell all callers that you will get back to them during those times.
■ Find out where the caller will be during those times.
■ In an emergency, tell them the doctor will call back immediately; but have your staff make sure it's really an emergency before interrupting you.

■ Make sure you *do* return calls during the times you've set. Otherwise, patients will lose confidence in you.

Cost

Do you feel our fees are fair? The cost of health care is of prime concern to consumers. If patients think your fees are too high, they might just go elsewhere.

Medical journals often contain articles about price not really being an object with patients. But inexorably, this is changing. In almost every survey, when patients are asked about the value of "price shopping" in seeking a physician, they almost always agree it's a good idea. How many are actually doing it? We don't yet know. But it's no longer looked upon as improper. And more and more patients are boldly asking, before making an appointment, "How much is it going to cost?"

What this means is that physicians should try to make patients see their services as "worth the price." The cost of care will be less of a marketing problem if you properly educate your patients about what they get for their money.

That's why you have to make yourself as accessible as possible, provide patients with information, satisfy their legitimate needs, and make sure your charges aren't out of line with those of your colleagues in the community.

Services

Question: Are you satisfied with the range of services we now offer? Physicians have traditionally tailored their services to their own personal and professional desires, with little regard for what patients want. "Doctor knows best." Right? Wrong! Because when it comes to the question of patients' needs, and even their desires, Doctor may have a lot to learn.

Much of what you may offer patients depends on your training as a physician. But additional services can often be provided if some thought is given to the subject. Here's an excellent example, taken from a four-member group of family physicians practicing in a rural Southern community.

Their survey showed patients were interested in routine dermatology care. A quick look at the demographics revealed the reason: Referrals for dermatology treatment were going to a doctor in a community more than 15 miles away. Patients don't want to travel far today. Remember? They want convenience and comfort. So what to do?

Well, a look at the marketing potential convinced them it was worth the price to send one of their number to a refresher course in dermatology, the costs to be paid by the practice. The expenditure proved justified. Though complicated cases are still referred, all routine dermatology is now handled within the group, and business has improved.

In an Eastern city, a surgeon found that many gallbladder and hernia patients also wanted him to take care of warts and moles. He'd always been bored by that type of office surgery. But he tried it. And the more he did it, the more he liked it—and his practice grew.

Patient desires for services changed the entire course of an internal medicine group in Chicago. At first they thought they should take on a general internist as a new partner. They surveyed their patients and uncovered an interest in arthritic services. So they began searching for a rheumatologist instead of a generalist. The decision paid off. When the specialist was added, he attracted numerous arthritis patients, who brought with them their additional medical needs.

Before beginning your survey, have a member of your staff pretest the questionnaire with a small number of patients on a one-to-one basis. The questions should be read to them to make sure there are no problems in understanding.

Once you've fashioned the questionnaire and conducted the survey, then what? Well, this is the part that generally brings a chorus of groans: Now you have to collect the responses, tabulate them in an orderly and uncomplicated fashion, use them to assess your strengths and weaknesses, and then prepare your marketing campaign. Take heart, it's not as onerous a task as it appears.

MAKING SENSE OF
YOUR SURVEY RESULTS
The more complicated the original survey, the more complicated the tabulation process will be. If the survey asked for subjective answers to all questions, you'll have to analyze each answer for its meaning—and that takes a lot of time. If your survey called for standard Yes or No answers, however, your job will be relatively easy.

The first step is to make up a tabulation sheet. You'll find the sample sheet in Appendix D a useful guide. Each question will have corresponding columns labeled Yes and No in which the number of responses for each will be recorded. For example:

Question	Yes	No
1.	218	371
2.	497	107
3.	258	252

The actual numbers of Yes and No responses mean very little. The percentage of each response is what counts. As a refresher for those who are rusty on such calculation, here's the way to compute it:

To get the percentage of Yes answers, divide the number of Yeses by the total of all Yeses and Noes. To get the percentage of No answers, divide the number of Noes by the total of all Yeses and Noes.

So, using the numbers from Question 1 above: The 218 Yeses plus 371 Noes total 589. The percentage of Yes answers to the question is 218 divided by 589, or 37 percent. The percentage of No answers is 371 divided by 589, or 63 percent.

Nothing could be simpler. Physicians, given their training in math, should find this procedure duck soup. But there's a psychological element in all this. Many doctors are looking for any excuse to dodge the job of surveying, and just such a minor roadblock as having to figure percentages can make them throw up their hands in frustration.

At one of our seminar workshops one physician became so agitated with the percentage explanation that he was almost ready to walk out. We asked what was wrong.

"I'm upset," he said, "because you're supposed to simplify my life, not complicate it! I was just beginning to think I might be able to do this survey with a minimum of time and effort. Now you're asking me to spend hours in calculating the results."

That wasn't what we were asking at all. Obviously, a busy doctor isn't going to have to do his own computations. Office staff can handle it, or bright young high school students can be hired to do it. A computer can do it, with a little help from human hands. Note that Chapter 16 deals with the marketing uses of the computer.

A Significant Response

The survey is now completed and the tabulation sheet filled out. But what have you got? Just a bunch of numbers. The next step is to determine which responses indicate probable trouble spots. For each question, you must identify what professional researchers call "the significant response." For our purposes, that would be the response that indicates a need for you to take action. Call it "the negative response," because it's the criticism that points to the problem. (A complete marketing plan will, of course, also accentuate and build on the positive responses you get from your patients, but for now let's address the problem side of the practice equation.)

Let's say you asked the question, "Is my office convenient for you to reach?" A heavy Yes response would mean that you have no problem in that area. Lucky you. No change required.

But suppose the response is an overwhelming No. Obviously, something is wrong with your location. That, then, is the significant response because it reveals a weakness in your practice. And that becomes part of the basis for your marketing plan.

The patient survey data analysis in Appendix D has the significant responses arranged in terms of ascending priorities according to the percentage of each response. If 75 percent of your patients are critical of some aspect of your practice, you'll obviously give a higher priority to correcting that situation than you would to a problem with only a 40 percent dissatisfaction.

In the final tabulation, place the appropriate percentage in the "significant response" column. The question: "Is my office convenient for you to reach?" That line on the completed tabulation sheet would look like this:

Question	Yes	No	% Yes	% No	Significant Response
9	100	400	20	80	80% No

Pick Marketing Priorities

Once you've tabulated your results, you can start the final phase of the research process—using those data to identify your strengths and weaknesses. If the right number of patients responded, you can conclude that their opinions pretty well represent the feelings of your practice as a whole.

As noted earlier, to set up your marketing plan, you must establish priorities and determine the order of the problems you'll attack.

During a marketing consultation with a three-member group in the South, their patient survey revealed that 10 percent were unhappy with the reception area. The most compulsive partner was ready to dash out and immediately change the whole decor.

It took a great deal of convincing to point out that 100 percent of their patients would never be completely satisfied, no matter what they did. If they had repainted with a different color, ordered new furniture, and installed wide-screen television and stereophonic sound, you can bet another 10 percent would hate it. On the other hand, no practice can afford to wait until everybody complains about the office, the staff, or whatever, before making changes. There has to be some point at which you take action or begin to lose patients. So you must have some rough guidelines on how to order your priorities. Here are our recommendations:

1. If less than 10 percent of those surveyed give a critical answer, a change generally isn't necessary.
2. If 10 to 25 percent are critical, you should take a close look at the situation, but you probably don't need to give it priority.

3. If 25 to 50 percent respond negatively, it deserves a medium priority.
4. If more than half your respondents think something is wrong, put the problem high on your list.
5. If more than 75 percent indicate dissatisfaction, you have a top-priority problem.

Negative Response	Priority Level
0 - 10%	None
10 - 25%	4
25 - 50%	3
50 - 75%	2
75 - 100%	1

Your next chore is to put your marketing-problem list in the same kind of priority order. Remember that each question addresses a particular issue, so your list should include the question and the information that the question analyzed, as follows:

Questions	Information Analyzed	Priority
3	Understanding specialty	1
12	Front office courtesy	1
14	Handling phone calls	1
6	Comfort of reception area	2
24	Health information	2
26	Time spent	3
33	Answering service	4

This survey is not, of course, *purely* concerned with negative reactions. It should also be used to identify your strengths. It's good for your practice, and for your ego, to make a list of areas that received less than 25 percent negative responses. You might be surprised at how satisfied, or nearly satisfied, your customers really are.

You can use that list of strengths to expand on your good points as you work on your marketing plan. Use it to make the rest of your personnel aware of their contribution to the practice. A warm pat on the back, or a little extra money in the pocket, for a job well done will go a long way toward gaining a staff's cooperation in improving your practice.

Appendix D gives you a completed and tabulated patient survey, with covering letter, directions for and results of data analysis, and responsive marketing priorities.

Summary _____ Our intent in this chapter was to alleviate some of your fears that a practice survey is a bottomless pit. We
hope we've succeeded. You should know now—if you didn't before—
that you must have the information the survey will bring, or you'll
simply continue to wander in the wilderness, making wild guesses at
what's wrong with your practice.

Reference

1. Peters TJ, Waterman RH: _In Search of Excellence._ New York: Harper &
   Row, 1982.

Resources

Boyd HW, et al: _Marketing Research: Text and Cases_, 5th ed. Homewood, IL:
Richard D. Irwin, 1981.
Bradford ES: _Bradford's Directory of Marketing Research Agencies and
Management Consultants in the United States and the World._ Fairfax, VA:
Bradford, 1984.
Kinnear T, Taylor JR: _Marketing Research: An Applied Approach._ New York:
McGraw-Hill, 1983.

CHAPTER 6

Put yourself in your patients' shoes

Until the very recent past, the public's attitude toward physicians was one of respect, bordering on reverence. Opinion polls consistently showed that physicians were respected and trusted by the American people.

But see what's happening now. In a survey conducted by the AMA in 1978, 87 percent of those polled expressed satisfaction with doctors. By 1983, the approval had dropped to 78 percent. If that trend continues for another 15 years, less than half our citizens will feel confidence in their doctors. Why have Americans started questioning the world's most respected health-care system? How has today's consumer of health care changed?

Many of the shifting attitudes parallel the shifting demographics of our society. Thirty years ago, America had a relatively stationary population. Most people were born, grew up, and worked in the same community all their lives. Allegiances to the "mom and pop" businesses were strong. Every family had its own favorite retail store, gas station—and doctor. Loyalty was important, and change was rare. But when our social trends changed, our loyalites began to take a beating.

THEY KEEP MOVING

In his book, *Megatrends*, John Naisbitt describes the trend as a shift from a centralized to a decentralized society.[1] For the first time since 1820, rural areas are growing faster than cities. The good news for doctors is that many physicians who settle in rural America find their practices thriving. The bad news is that the American public is moving out of the cities as fast as the physicians are moving in. *(See Fig. 6-A)*

As America shifts from a stable industrial society to a mobile informational society, large businesses are decentralizing their offices. This creates more frequent moves, particularly for employees climbing the corporate ladder. A large segment of our population moves every three to five years. The latest census showed that as many as one in five Americans moves *every* year. In our affluence, we have become what John Steinbeck said of the depression poor: "a migrant people."

In a small suburban practice in the Midwest, 30 percent of the patients who left in a six-month period were in the 30 to 45 age group. They left town because they'd been transferred. In a survey we conducted for the Arizona Medical Association, 50 percent of the patients had been with their current doctor less than six years.

Those trends play a great part in consumers' attitudes toward physicians. It's hard to be loyal to one doctor when you know you'll be moving on in a few years. People are not quick to connect with a physician when they move into a new community. Many wait until they get sick before finding a doctor in a phone book, or putting themselves at the mercy of the local emergency room for a referral. Also, realizing that they'll not be with a particular physician for long, people are more willing to shop around. You can see the tremendous implications this has for the marketing of private physicians' services.

CHANGING MOVEMENTS

America's social changes play an equally important role in altering the attitudes of patients. Let's take a look at four major movements:

Health Rights

In 1944, people began to look at health care differently when President Franklin D. Roosevelt asked Congress for an "economic bill of rights." That bill, finally passed under the Truman Administration, included the right of all citizens to adequate health care and protection from the "economic fear" of illness. The affirmation of the power of any citizen to place demands on the medical-delivery system became known as the Patient's Bill of Rights.

Figure 6-A
DEMOGRAPHIC TRENDS

Centralized	Decentralized
Stationary	Migratory
Urban	Rural

In 1972, the American Hospital Association adopted a series of consumer-advocacy reforms that included the rights to informed consent, to considerate and respectful care, and to refuse treatment within the extent permitted by law. That document forever changed the feeling that patients had to take whatever health care they were given, without question or input. Patients no longer feel bound to an unswerving, reverent, and grateful attitude toward all doctors.

The Women's Movement _____ For many years the major consumers of health care have been women. They are involved with physician services at about twice the rate of men. Much of that has been due to their roles as mothers. Women, as the primary caretakers of children, had the job of taking them to the doctor. And because most women were homemakers, they had more time to go to the doctor themselves.

The awful truth is that during the 19th and early 20th centuries women were brainwashed into believing that they were "the weaker sex" and that their "female problems" made it necessary for them to seek more medical attention. But as women rightfully gained more confidence in themselves, they became more aggressive in finding physicians who respected them as people, and as women. They no longer fell for the old "time of the month" dodge. They began to demand real answers to their problems.

Today, more and more women have their own successful careers. They're finding it difficult to find time to go to the doctor, particularly if the doctor is not easily accessible. The changing roles of women have, therefore, weakened the link of the family with traditional and routine medical care.

A contributing factor has been the development of vaccines against virtually every childhood ailment, thus drastically reducing the number of times that mother—or father—must take the children to the doctor.

This transformation of women from passive receivers into aggressive seekers has had a big impact on the health-care scene. Physicians who fail to take those changes into consideration are buying themselves trouble.

Self-care

In the 1960s, Americans began to be disenchanted with the traditional wisdom that medicine could solve all their health problems. Some attributed the change to medicine's failure to make more dramatic breakthroughs in finding a cure for cancer. Others point to medicine's apparent lack of interest in nutrition. Regardless of the reason, Americans now place a much greater importance on taking care of themselves.

Look at how the new emphasis on self-care has affected us. At least 100 million Americans are now exercising regularly. Smoking is down some 25 percent. The number of health food stores increased almost seven-fold, from 1,200 in 1968 to 8,300 in 1981. Those trends contribute to the overall health potential of the American public, yet they also signal an end to the belief that physicians know all there is to know about health. The self-care movement has opened a Pandora's Box of nonphysicians who provide services that were once in the traditional physician's domain.

Patients don't run to a doctor for advice on nutrition, exercise, or even the diagnosis of many medical problems. Consumers can now perform tests at home for pregnancy, diabetes, and even certain types of cancer. One New York research firm estimates the sales of self-diagnosis kits as topping $100 million in 1990. Almost every month, a new self-test appears on the market.

The concept that patients are responsible enough to diagnose their own ills also embraces the feeling that they can pick the types of specialists they need. The idea of self-referral is resulting in more and more limited specialists receiving calls directly from patients who have decided, on their own, that they need one particular kind of care. The general public wholeheartedly wants a self-help health system, not one dominated by doctors.

Prevention has become the watchword. Americans are giving more attention to stopping illness before it starts. Unfortunately, the emphasis physicians place on prevention seems to lag behind that of the general public, and as new organizations have catered to this demand, prevention has rapidly become a growth industry.

The Holistic Movement

Holistic health care deals with the body, mind, and emotions as inseparable units. It has gained a large following among those who believe health is determined by more than physicals, regular checkups, tests, and drugs. They believe that the interaction of various facets of one's entire being creates a state of wellness. Many feel that medicine's apparent—or real—lack of concern about nutrition, and its emphasis on tests and drugs, have played into the hands of the holistic movement. You've probably heard this criticism: "Doctors don't know anything about nutrition." Well, many Americans feel that if physicians aren't experts in nutrition, then they can't be experts in wellness. As a result, many medical patients are being lost to holistic practitioners.

CHANGING DEMANDS

Several months ago, a seminar group was asked if patients choose a doctor on the basis of quality. The immediate response was, "Of course!"

But when asked *how* patients could judge quality, the group remained silent. Then, one by one, they came up with the standard answers: "The medical school attended, the residency training, years in practice, continuing education credits."

The audience seemed relieved when told that surveys indicated that the public did, indeed, choose physicians on the basis of perceived quality. But silence fell again when the rest of the findings were announced: The American public doesn't really have much basis for being able to judge quality in a physician. Yes, they've been told that the US has the best health-care system in the world. True. But in selling that to the public, we've inadvertently sold the idea that *all* practitioners in the system are quality physicians.

As has been pointed out, patients use surrogate perceptions to judge the differences between your quality and that of your competitors. That is, they judge your environment, your staff, your nurses, and the

Figure 6-B
INFLUENCES ON PATIENTS

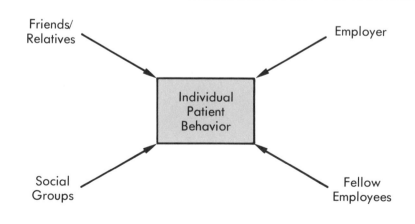

amount of convenience, comfort, information, and understanding you give them. And they are influenced by the opinions of others (see Fig. 6-B), which are generally also based on those surrogate perceptions.

Here's a look at the all-important factors that determine their choice:

Convenience

Banks give us automatic tellers. Gas stations give us self-service pumps. Supermarkets and other stores stay open around the clock. The whole fast-food industry was founded on the premise that Americans want to eat what they want, where they want, when they want, and as fast as they want.

Convenience is the new name of the game. If you don't give that to the consumer, you may as well fold your tent and move out of the way. Until the late 1970s, health care was one of the few service industries that didn't tailor its service to its customers. Private physicians are still suffering from this failure. You need look only at the success of the freestanding primary-care centers to see what the public wants. More than 20 million people have used these facilities, not because they offer higher quality care than the private practitioner, but because they are convenient.

Why should a patient take time off from work, perhaps lose part of a day's pay, to see a doctor when he can be cared for at a convenience clinic on the way home at night?

Health Education

The four areas of greatest informational and educational interest to the public are sports, weather, health, and sex—not necessarily in that order. Americans have a seemingly unquenchable thirst for health-related information about diabetes, blood pressure, arthritis, heart disease, nutrition, and exercise. Magazines, newspapers, radio, and television all recognize the need and cater to it with a mass of health-related articles and programs. Unfortunately, the quality is not always the best.

Physicians who provide good, solid health information for their patients have a leg up on improving their market.

Medical Information

There is a difference between health education and medical information. Health education relates broadly to diseases, nutrition, and the like. Medical information provides knowledge of a patient's particular medical problem.

Patients are asking more questions. They don't always accept the doctor's opinion as gospel. They're asking why certain tests are needed; how much things cost; if this or that is really necessary for a diagnosis. They no longer take prescriptions blindly. They inquire about side effects; interactions with other drugs; generic substitutions. Do you have any idea how many of your patients own a *Physicians' Desk Reference* or *The Merck Manual?*

Patients are becoming very knowledgeable consumers, and some physicians aren't handling their questions very well. Some resent these "self-taught" patients. That's a foolish reaction. Be glad they're interested. An informed patient is a much easier patient to work with in the long run. There's nothing worse than the fear, phobias, and resistance brought on by ignorance.

Time and Attention
Years ago, patients were grateful for any time the doctor gave them. Now the consumer feels his or her time is as valuable as the doctor's—which it is. Again, let us remind you that "time" spent with the patient is not important quantitatively, only qualitatively. The ability to communicate is the doctor's key.

When you're doing a poor job of getting through to the patient, spending a lot of time does little good. But if you can communicate well, with a caring attitude, a minute becomes golden. So, improve your communications skills as much as possible.

Partnership in Health
In today's automated, computerized society, a lot of people find it hard to achieve an identity. Many of the social movements of the 1970s and 1980s were and are attempts to be recognized as more than a number, and this search for identity includes the doctor-patient relationship. Remember the jokes about patients being referred to as "the liver problem" or "the kidney?" No more. American consumers see nothing funny about that. They demand to be treated as individuals, not as diseases. What's more, they want to be treated as partners in their health care. And they're right.

Their input can make our health-care system work better. We're not talking about making diagnoses. We're talking about the patient's right to question and voice opinions about the care and treatment of his or her own body. *(See Fig. 6-C)*

Almost all successful executives achieve their goals by exercising their ability to listen to and relate to their customers and employees. Japan, for example, has achieved the world's highest productivity partially through "quality circles." All employees have direct input

Figure 6-C
PATIENT WANTS AND NEEDS

- Convenience
- Health Education
- Medical Information
- More Quality Time
- Partnership in Health

into calling attention to and solving problems. Management and labor, in effect, form a partnership.

That's what doctor and patient must do. The physician who keeps patients at a distance and ignores their potential input does so today at risk of a shrinking patient base.

Summary

The bedrock of the marketing concept is consumer orientation, and the first step is to identify the consumer's wants and needs. This chapter has presented some of the reasons why today's health-care consumer differs from the consumer of 20, or even 10 years ago. It has also identified some of the wants and needs of today's consumers as discovered through marketing research. Your job now is to devise ethical ways to satisfy your patients so they and you end up in a "win-win" situation.

Reference

Naisbitt J: *Megatrends*. New York: Warner Books, 1982.

Resources

The American Health Care System. Chicago: American Medical Association, 1982.
Brown SW: Consumer and physician attitudes toward physicians' services, *Arizona Medicine*, Vol. 37, No. 1, 33-36.
Engel JF, Blackwell R: *Consumer Behavior*, 4th edition. Hinsdale, Illinois: The Dryden Press, 1982.
Howard JA, Sheth JN: *The Theory of Buyer Behavior*. New York: John Wiley & Sons, 1969.
Maslow AH: *Motivation and Personality*. New York: Harper & Row, 1954.

CHAPTER 7

You have more markets than you realize

When toothpaste was being sold 50 years ago, there were relatively few brands, and they were marketed for only one purpose—to clean teeth. At least, that's what the manufacturers thought. The market was seen as one homogeneous mass.

But as more and more brands appeared and competition intensified, a search began to find other reasons for using toothpaste. Market researchers came up with three categories of needs or wants: People wanted to prevent cavities. They wanted whiter teeth. They desired sweeter breath. Suddenly, the market was heterogeneous—"segmented" into groups based on similar wants and needs. *(See Fig. 7-A)*

So the various virtues of toothpaste were advertised through specific ads aimed at one or more of these groups. Ipana, for example, pledged to give us "the smile of beauty!" Until the market survey was made, no one thought to promise that toothpaste would make one beautiful.

Manufacturers not only upped the cleaning power; they improved the taste, sought approvals from the dental profession

Figure 7-A
THE TOOTHPASTE MARKET

1925
Homogeneous Demand

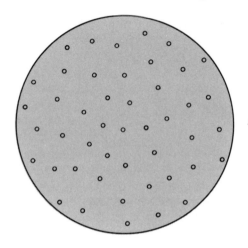

All Users Desired Clean Teeth

1985
Heterogeneous Demand

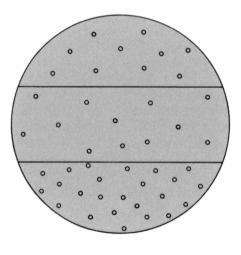

Users Desiring Whiter Teeth

Users Desiring Fresh Breath

Users Desiring Cavity Prevention

and testing organizations, and endorsements from celebrities. Look at the results today.

Another classic example of market segmentation affecting product development was Henry Ford's "Model T." It was a mass-produced product, each black car exactly like every other. But with market segmentation, automakers developed a full line of differently designed cars, with different features, and painted in different colors. And what a difference it made. Today we have compacts, subcompacts, convertibles, hatchbacks, two doors, four doors, four cylinders, six cylinders, eight cylinders—each variation with its own appeal to some consumer group. Even within the same auto company, divisions compete against one another. For example: Chevrolet, Pontiac, Oldsmobile, Buick, and Cadillac—all General Motors' divisions—often vie for the same customers.

WHICH PATIENTS DO YOU WANT?

Competition in health care also demands segmentation of the market because, although you may know that you want more patients, you may not be sure which ones you want or how to appeal to them.

Let's look at some of the information you've already collected from demographic, practice, patient, and personal surveys. As you review your findings, note any areas you should be pursuing. One physician had always been interested in dermatology. When he found that 45 percent of his patients would prefer to come to him for their skin care, rather than go to the specialist he'd been recommending, he took courses to upgrade his skills in that specialty. His new talents made him unique among providers of primary care in that area. Dermatology became his special niche.

Or let's suppose 35 percent of your patients would like you to provide dietary counseling. A quick survey might show an absence of other good facilities to furnish that service in your area. If you were to set up an office-based dietary service, you could probably broaden your market quite easily.

Segment Current Patients

What you're trying to do is to divide your practice according to areas of common interest, goals, needs, wants, and various other characteristics.

By Age. While this factor provides the greatest potential for the field of primary care, even a narrower specialty practice can find age groups for which distinctive needs and wants can be identified. One of the greatest potentials is in the geriatric group. With the changes taking place in Medicare reimbursement, a wide range of services for older people may soon be lacking. Examples: home health care, day care, nutritional counseling, blood pressure and diabetic screening. The doctor who can effectively provide such services for the elderly won't have a shortage of patients.

By Disease. Many doctors limit themselves by treating patients as a homogeneous group. They use the same methods in treating diabetes and heart disease as they do with COPD. They tend to overlook the specific problems inherent in each disease. If you singled out the diabetics within your practice, for example, you could provide specific times for their blood sugar checks, give training in diabetic diets, and conduct classes on special skin care, since diabetes increases the incidence of skin infection.

Take hypertensives. One of the most critical problems for this group of patients is compliance. Providing a strategy that would help them do the things necessary for their improvement and survival would be well accepted. Most patients want to comply, if shown how to do it with a minimum of inconvenience (see Chapter 15).

By Services Desired. While conducting a practice audit in Atlanta, we found that one of the specific services patients wanted was family counseling. Those who needed it felt they'd like to receive it from their primary physician. But could he provide it?

The decision had to be based on his level of expertise, the cost-effectiveness for the practice, and the number of patients who would be interested. He finally decided that the best move was to hire a clinical psychologist to join the practice several afternoons a week on a fee-for-service basis.

The physician didn't make any money directly from the venture, but within six months he had an amazing increase in the number of new patients. Many of them said they were attracted to the practice because of the new psychological service, and they remained in the practice for the rest of their health care.

Still another doctor took advantage of the new emphasis on women and their health needs to develop services that would appeal to them. A major element was the creation of a clinic to treat premenstrual syndrome.

Segment Potential Patients

Obviously, it's difficult to devise a strategy broad enough to attract a homogeneous population. Our competitive medical environment has created a situation not unlike that of the toothpaste makers. We must be able to identify specific groups with specific needs.

Your potential patients can be split up in much the same way that we divided your current patients—according to age, disease, and need. You can also differentiate by demographics.

By Age. A young internist conducted a personal and practice survey and decided to see more geriatric patients. He had special training in gerontology, but for him to jump on his marketing horse and begin galloping before he knew where he was going would only lead him to grief.

We first suggested that he plot his potential patients according to age. If special demographic information were translated into where the aging population of the community was centered, he could then see where to target his marketing efforts.

To find sections heavy with older people, he was asked to get a community map and a supply of colored pins. First, he had to identify the center of the older residential areas, pinpointing all retirement centers and homes. Then, we had him mark the districts with the oldest registered voters. All this information was easily obtained from various civic and business agencies.

Once the map was completed, it was easy to see that the doctor's then current practice population was well outside areas with heavy concentrations of the elderly. To reach these older people, he conducted an outreach marketing program, beginning with speeches to civic and retiree groups in the target areas. After he did that, the geriatric element in his practice began to grow, almost immediately.

By Disease. There are two ways to classify your potential practice area according to specific diseases:

First, many diseases orient themselves to community screening programs. For example: More than 20 percent of any population likely has undetected hypertension. Since a portion of those people aren't under the care of any physician, that portion represents potential patients. The task for the physician is to identify them through ethical marketing programs, such as free blood-pressure screening in the office, and through public-education programs on the importance of early detection. Patients who have no physician are likely to stay with the doctor who identifies their disease.

Second, many doctors conduct surveys to find patients with particular diseases they want to treat. One example is the physician, noted earlier, who had an interest in premenstrual syndrome. She reached her own female patients and offered them services to match their needs by creating a PMS clinic. But if she had also used ethical mar-

Figure 7-B
MARKETING RESEARCH RESOURCES

Agency	Information Provided
Cooperative Extension Service Rural Development Offices State University Local Census Bureau	County statistics, including economic, agricultural, population, and public assistance programs
State Hospital Association	Local hospitals, allied personnel, and physician distribution
Local Hospitals	Many gather demographic information for their own marketing purposes
Health System Agencies	Both demographic and manpower information plus future projections of need
State Human Resources/Health Department	Vital statistics on primary care clinics and other funded sources of medical care
State Licensing Boards	Physician-manpower statistics
Local Chamber of Commerce Better Business Bureau Business Licensing Board	Local business trends and information on county development and growth potential
County Office of Building Permits Commercial Real Estate Board	Present and future trends in housing and new growth potential
County Medical Association State Medical Association AMA State and National Specialty Societies	Statistics on physician distribution and patient-physician ratios
County Office for the Aging Local Meals-on-Wheels Local Retirement Homes Local Medicare/Medicaid offices	Target population of over-65 group, including distribution, health-care needs, and projections on growth
State/Local School Boards	Statistics and estimates on school enrollment

keting tools to identify other women in her community in need of those services, she would have had a fine target market.

Note, please, that this sort of reaching out not only improves a physician's marketing position; it also improves the quality of health care delivered.

By Services. Many doctors identify areas of personal interest that can be translated into services that meet the needs of particular patient groups. A young orthopedist, for example, found himself in the middle of a highly competitive market. A personal evaluation revealed that he had a specific interest in sports medicine. A quick look at community trends showed that he was in an area of young people, with many amateur sports teams—an ideal environment into which he could introduce his interest in sports medicine.

He singled out the sports enthusiasts of the area by offering himself as a team doctor. His offer was quickly accepted by several organizations. He also appealed directly to the coaches by offering to give talks on conditioning and on care of athletic injuries. The coaches responded enthusiastically and became an unofficial but dependable referral system.

So "external market segmentation"—looking for groups of new patients—allows physicians to find market niches and to concentrate their marketing efforts on identifying and attracting a specific group of patients. Caution: Don't try to construct a single complicated plan to embrace all those potential patients out there. Identify specific markets and develop a separate plan for each.

Segment Other Sources
While identification—segmentation—of current and potential patient populations will probably be your most productive method, other local sources can also be segmented. Here are two:

Industry. A floundering primary-care group was located in a heavily industrial area in the Northeast. In looking for ways to expand their market, the physicians realized they had been concentrating solely on patients. But why couldn't the business community also be segmented into target markets? We asked if they were interested in occupational medicine. They saw no reason they couldn't develop their expertise along that line.

A quick survey of several local industries revealed that many had no established physician or practice to handle their workers' compensation needs. So the group devised a marketing plan to provide those services to two of the larger plants in the area. They scheduled a meeting with executives and took them on a tour of their medical complex. Within several weeks they were seeing three to four workers per day. They now report that several other businesses have contacted them.

Referring Physicians. During one of our presentations, a surgeon asked how concentrating on specific target areas could benefit a practice that relies largely on referrals. Our reply: "Why not single out the referring physicians?" The surgeon did just that, first making a list of all his current referring doctors. He then broke the list down into six-month referral patterns for each doctor. Object: To see which had slowed down or increased their rates of referrals. Those who had stopped referring patients, or who were referring fewer of them, could then be informally contacted to ask the reason for the decline. The surgeon also developed a second list of potential referring physicians he could contact through various channels.

Summary
The goal of segmentation is to identify the particular needs of specific groups within your market. It's a way to find and enter the special niche in the marketplace that you, and perhaps only you, can fill. In short, segmentation identifies the targets of your marketing plan.

PART III

YOUR MARKETING PLANS AND PROGRAMS

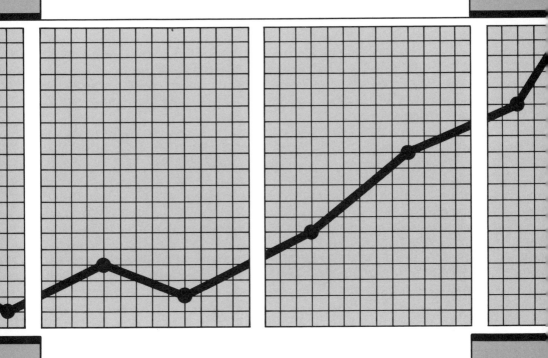

CHAPTER 8

You've got to have a marketing plan

You've already identified, researched, and analyzed your practice problems and opportunities. You've also identified your target markets. It's time now to consider how to develop a marketing plan to put your practice into the best position.

THE FOUR CORNERS OF MARKETING

Four factors must be considered before laying out your marketing plan: your consumers' needs and wants, coordination of your practice to carry out the program, the necessity of using ethical methods, and the need for executing your plan in a cost-effective manner.

1. Consumer Orientation

After reviewing the data and identifying what the customer is looking for, sit back and look at your practice through the patient's eyes. You must be brutally honest with your appraisals, or you'll end up with an unrealistic, unreliable marketing plan. For objectivity, it might be wise to have someone outside the practice review your appraisal. A good choice would be another professional—possibly an attorney, since lawyers are trained to observe and analyze just as doctors are.

2. Integrated Effort

All members of the practice must be committed to the marketing philosophy. The physician who likes to remain relatively isolated from colleagues and staff may have to come out of the shell a bit. Staff meetings must be held to explain the marketing needs and goals. Of prime importance: The basic principles must be agreed upon by your staff so everyone doesn't end up pulling in different directions.

3. Social Responsibility

A physician's responsibilities and ethics transcend both the marketplace and the quest for survival. Your first responsibility is still to provide high-quality, cost-effective care that's in the best interest of the patient. Who can argue with that? And when the basics of a good marketing plan have been reviewed, you'll see that the planning actually reinforces and enhances those socially responsible principles.

4. Profit Motivation

When marketing was first introduced to the world of the physician, the word "profit" often was left out of the presentations. Many felt that doctors would be criticized for even discussing profit, and especially for teaching principles that could be viewed as merely profit-oriented.

The days of "the rich doctor who lives on the hill" are just about over. But there's no reason the doctor, like anyone else, shouldn't earn a fair profit. Why shouldn't the doctor be concerned when income declines under pressures of the competitive environment? Entrepreneurs of the health-care industry certainly don't shy from trying to generate a profit. Why shouldn't the doctor have the right to a reasonably comfortable economic situation? Practice costs, which include educational expenses, must be recovered. And beyond overt outlay, there must be decent recompense for the huge time commitment and the emotional and physical stress of practicing medicine.

No matter how the physician may justify the profit made, the ultimate criterion has to be whether the marketing plan meets the wants and needs of the consumer in a cost-effective manner. Fail in this area, and the whole structure may collapse.

Numerous studies have shown that the public doesn't begrudge a physician's income unless they feel it greatly exceeds a reasonable profit. Of course, the definition of reasonable will differ. But so long as medicine is perceived as cost-contained, cost-effective, and as adequately satisfying society's needs for health care, the American public seems unlikely to disapprove of doctors making profit.

PRACTICE MISSION

During a recent seminar we asked, "What business are you in?" It caught the participants off guard. Many of the physicians seemed confused, wondering if they'd heard correctly. Their answers were both revealing and troubling:

"I'm in the business of medicine."

"I'm in the business of doing surgery."

"I'm in the business of seeing patients."

Wrong, wrong, wrong. To understand why, let's look at our railroads—the dominant business of the late 1800s, and one that continued to flourish as a major industry well into this century. After World War II, however, the once thriving giant almost faded from the scene. Early leaders of the industry were convinced that railroads would dominate American business for a long time. Myopically, they viewed their business as "railroading." That worked so long as there was no real competition in transporting people and goods. But as new alternatives emerged, America eventually lost interest in railroads as the primary means of transportation, and the industry began to run out of steam.

Belatedly, railroad executives realized that they were actually in the highly competitive "transportation" business. This different orientation allowed many companies to change with the times and to move people and goods by the most appropriate methods of transportation—not just the railroad. To think of themselves simply as "railroaders" was too constricting.

So, Doctor, "What business are you in?" Your answer should be, "I'm in the business of satisfying the wants and needs of my patients. I'm in the business of providing the highest quality of health care available in a compassionate, cost-effective manner." Taking that perspective, you're in much less danger of looking at your marketing strategies so narrowly that you fail to meet your basic obligations to patients.

STRATEGIC AND TACTICAL PLANNING

In military terms, strategic planning is long-range; tactical planning is immediate. In like manner, marketing can involve both long-range and immediate planning.

Tactical plans are designed to handle the most urgent problems during the first two years, while the stage is being set for solutions that will take longer to accomplish. The short-range plan, however, isn't simply an element of the long-range plan; it's self-contained and should be directed toward all goals of the marketing plan.

The long-range plan covers up to 20 years. It's very difficult to convince physicians to project their thinking that far into the future. Most are oriented to the short term, and tend to concentrate on "quick fix" plans. But doctors can and must extend their planning horizon to at least three years. Distinguishing between short- and long-range goals isn't difficult. Try your hand at the following:

- Improve the quality of the staff.
- Provide better scheduling for shorter waiting times.
- Anticipate an influx of new physicians.
- Increase current patient load by 25 percent.

The first two goals are short-range because they'd have an immediate impact on the practice. The latter two goals, however, will have greater impact further down the road.

YOUR FOUR MARKETING OPTIONS

Four basic options are open to you in considering the objectives of your marketing planning. *(See Fig. 8-A)*

1. Entrenchment

You can elect to draw your wagons into a circle and direct all your marketing efforts toward retaining the patients you have. This "entrenchment philosophy" is exemplified by a physician in a large Northern industrial state who was faced with increasing competition. After analyzing the situation, he decided to concentrate on satisfying the patients he had, rather than attracting new ones. While not designed to do so, this approach may serve to expand your practice by generating a number of referrals from your current patients.

2. Market Development

This involves making potential patients aware of your practice. It deals primarily with the promotional aspects of marketing. Its success, however, depends on the strengths of the present practice, and it may require a significant financial commitment. Market development will work, if your present strengths far outweigh weaknesses, and if your current practice meets the wants and needs of the potential patients.

Figure 8-A
MARKETING OPTIONS

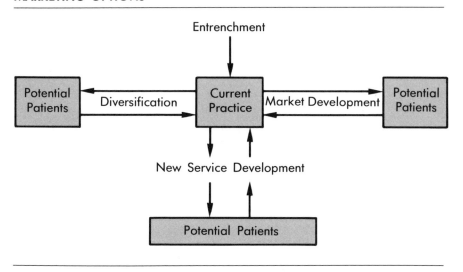

3. New Service Development
You can add new dimensions to a practice by changing the present pattern of services, or by adding new ones to make it more satisfying and attractive to both present and potential patients. A physician who attends seminars on the problems of treating adolescents, and then adds this service to the practice, is utilizing a new service approach. In most cases, it improves patient satisfaction. This approach pays off in terms of referrals stimulated by satisfied patients. Beware, however. If the new services are concentrated too much on the needs of potential patients, while not meeting the needs of present patients, the plan could backfire.

4. Diversification
Remember the young orthopedist, mentioned earlier, who emphasized sports medicine in his practice? He's an example of a doctor who elected to diversify into a new service and gain new patients via some special promotional efforts. If current data are correct, practices that diversify stand the greatest chance of expanding their markets.

In reality, most marketing plans combine various elements of each of those four options. Trying to survive by sticking exclusively with one may result in too narrow a plan for both short- and long-range success. The option—or options—you choose will depend on your

Figure 8-B
THE 4-P MARKETING MIX

- Product/Service
- Price
- Place/Accessibility
- Promotion/Communication

practice setting and goals, the resources available, and the time needed to achieve the goals.

IN THE MARKETING MIX
Marketing strategy means getting the right product or service to the right place at the right time and for the right price. It must include consideration of product/service, price, place/accessibility, and promotion. A successful marketing strategy must emphasize and interrelate all elements of this "marketing mix."

Henry Ford provides a good lesson in not putting all the Ps into his market basket. He was best known as a production genius. He was also an astute marketing strategist, who was first to see the potential profit in a low-priced car for the mass market. Before he came on the scene, the market was small and specialized because manufacturers produced cars only for the very wealthy. *(Figs. 8-B and 8-C)*

Figure 8-C
FROM MODEL-T TO MARKET MIX

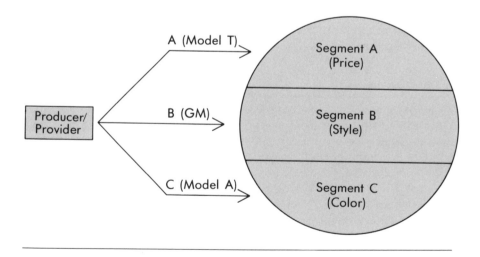

It's ironic, therefore, that Ford later failed to see the need for diversity in automobiles. And so, in the 1920s, he was still offering his mass-produced car "in any color, as long as it's black."

Along came Alfred Sloan Jr., the man who helped create General Motors. He cashed in on Ford's standpat attitude. Sloan saw a market with several distinct segments based on desire for the product, price, accessibility, and the promotional efforts required to sell the idea to the public. So GM developed a new line of cars, adding a variety of colors and stylings, even though it meant raising prices.

The idea wasn't immediately successful, but it caught up with Henry Ford in the late 1920s, forcing him to close down his assembly plants and revamp his strategy. Ford's answer was the Model A, in various colors.

And so *your* marketing strategy should also be concerned with the development of a marketing mix designed to reach definite segments of your present and potential consumers.

Summary

The new, competitive atmosphere not only offers your patients a broader, more available set of options in health care, but it encourages you to define and develop your services. To take advantage of the opportunities, you must become more aggressive in your approach to the marketplace.

CHAPTER 9

Making your services more appealing

Now that your research is completed, market segments given priorities, and marketing goals set, each goal must be analyzed in terms of the four Ps of the marketing mix—Product, Price, Place, and Promotion. Each P will be discussed in a chapter of its own, beginning with Product.

To put the entire marketing mix into perspective, you must first understand the relationship of your *product* or *services* to your marketing plan. To do this, you have to consider the basis of all commerce—the exchange process.

THE EXCHANGE PROCESS: PRODUCT AND VALUE

In traditional marketing, the exchange process is defined as "the offering of a product...in exchange for something of value."[1] Both parties—whether a retailer and a shopper, or a doctor and a patient—should benefit from the exchange. *(See Fig. 9-A)*

A product or service may be defined from either the producer's or the consumer's point of view. But it's the consumer's view

Figure 9-A
THE EXCHANGE PROCESS

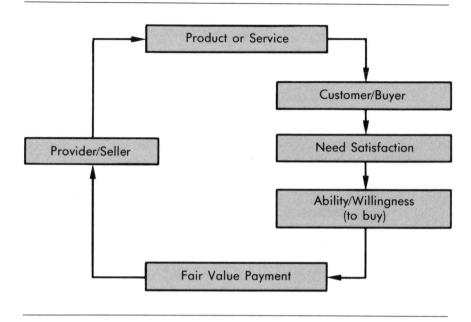

that counts. And the result of not recognizing that is illustrated by what happened some years ago when the DuPont corporation attempted to introduce a synthetic product called Corfam as a substitute for leather.

From a technological standpoint, Corfam had many advantages, including durability and the quality of snapping back into its original shape. DuPont was so convinced of the product's ultimate success that large amounts of money were invested in its development and promotion. Consumers, however, were more interested in style and comfort than in durability. Leather, though less durable, had a better appearance and conformed to the foot, which Corfam did not.

The product failed, not because of any technical fault, but because the producer failed to find out what the consumer really wanted. It's a lesson that can teach physicians a lot about interacting with patients.

**Selling Yourself
and Your Services** ————————— Like most physicians, you probably don't think of yourself as "selling" a service or product. Just the thought may make you flinch. Yet you certainly don't hesitate to say

that you're "providing" or "offering" health care—a service, and in a sense, also a product. While you may think that the owner of your favorite restaurant is "selling" food, he may say he's "providing" or "offering" meticulous service and exquisite delicacies. In the marketplace of health care, the concept of "selling" your services and of patients "buying" them is both acceptable and realistic.

Below are some examples of the various forms that physicians' services may take. We've selected the most obvious to show how many areas of your practice you can involve in your marketing plans.

A pediatrician offers examinations, physicals, immunizations, the prescribing of appropriate medicines, and 24-hour-a-day availability in emergencies. The last is vital. While an ill adult will wait for a doctor, it's a rare parent who will tolerate a delay in medical attention for a child.

An obstetrician is selling his expertise in the care of expectant mothers and unborn children via prenatal visits, tests, and deliveries.

A family physician's services involve the broad field of primary care. This breaks down into various evaluations, physicals, shots, counseling, and health education.

A radiologist's products are expert evaluations of films, recommendations of proper testing, and special radiologic procedures.

As you can see, every element of the profession has its own services and products to offer, and it's important to understand this variety in formulating marketing strategies.

In one of our seminars, a physician was asked to explain what his product was. After some thought, he said it was "the care I provide." But when asked to explain what that care included, he confessed he'd never sat down and tried to list the things he did for his patients.

How are you going to know what to change or improve if you don't have a handle on all you do? Try listing everything that you offer patients. The following categories should be helpful in itemizing your product and services:

1. Product-Physician (You)
Education
Training
Expertise
Experience

2. Primary Services
Examinations
Physicals
Acute Care
Chronic Care

3. Ancillary Services
Counseling
Testing
Therapies
Evaluations

4. Business Services
Appointments
Financial Assistance
Insurance Assistance

5. Other Services
Physical Plant
Office Atmosphere
Staff Support

Once the list is completed, show it to your staff, and perhaps to several patients to see if you've left anything out. Your list probably won't agree completely with what your patients think of your practice. (Keep those Corfam shoes in mind when making your list.) Giving patients a product that *you* think is beneficial, without considering what *they* think, is not only costly; it's poor marketing.

The Patient's View

As noted earlier, patients see you as offering much more than the obvious health care you think of as your primary, and perhaps only, service. They define your practice by their total experience with you, your staff, and your office. Their definition is formed by at least six impressions:

- During the pre-visit phone call.
- Upon arrival at your office.
- In the reception area and examining rooms.
- While with you.
- Departing from your office.
- Contact after the visit.

The dramatically different views often seen by doctor and patient can be likened to two people looking into opposite ends of a telescope. You simply have to look through your patients' end to see their perspective. *(See Fig. 9-B)*

Your Physical Plant. We'll never forget the shock of arriving at a very highly recommended restaurant in Atlanta some years ago. The place was nothing more than a shabby hole in the wall with dirt on the floor. We turned right around and walked out. The surroundings were simply too offensive. They were surrogate indicators of the expected quality of the food.

As we happily learned later, we were wrong. The food truly was of gourmet quality. So why the shabbiness and dirtiness? The restaurant had so much business it didn't need elegant decor or a clean floor. But how many people have walked out, as we did, basing their decisions on those first impressions?

The restaurant owners could get away with their attitude, not only because of their food—they also had virtually no competition in that area. The vast majority of physicians today can't operate with the restaurant owners' attitude, no matter how good they are as clinicians. A case in point:

When we were asked to look at the marketing problems of a struggling practice in the Northwest, it took about two minutes to find the main weakness. The reception area was a disaster: The chairs were as comfortable as medieval torture racks, the corners of the room were encrusted with dirt, the lighting was dim, and the ventilation was nonexistent. The whole atmosphere was depressing. Then we met the doctors. Both were attractively groomed and looked more like executives than physicians. The contrast was striking.

When asked about the condition of their office, they laughed, saying they'd been planning some renovation for years, but had never gotten around to it. "You know," said one, "interest rates are so high and the costs just aren't worth it."

"So what are your practice problems?" we asked.

"Several new physicians have moved into the area. We've been here for years, and until now we've had all we could handle. But this new competition has cut into our practice quite a bit."

One of the doctors invited us to dinner that evening. Her house and furnishings were magnificent, the dinner elegant, and the atmosphere first class. We wondered how she could put so much emphasis on comfort and convenience at home, yet pay so little attention to them in her office.

It wasn't by coincidence that the new physicians in town had set up a very attractive physical plant. Potential patients were pleased by the atmosphere, and once there, they stayed.

Patients place great importance on the external appearance of your product. That includes everything in your reception area. (It's always "the reception area," never "the waiting room." You don't want to imply that people will have to wait.)

Be sure to have light, airy, pleasant surroundings. The reception area should be air conditioned, have plenty of good reading materials, and perhaps a TV or pleasant background music, according to your patients' taste. This, incidentally, would be an excellent inquiry for your patient survey: Would you like TV or music in our office? If music, what kind?

One of the best ways to start is to spend some time in your reception area. At one of our recent seminars, a doctor's spouse commented that her husband entered his office through a rear door and hadn't been in his reception area in more than five years! Be sure not to let that happen to you.

Take a hard look at your area. Check the comfort of the chairs, the nature and dates of the reading material. Is the lighting too dim? Too glaring? Are the walls fresh and bright, or soiled and in need of paint? Ask yourself if you'd like having to sit there for a half hour, especially if you're waiting to find out what your illness is, and if it can be treated. Here's a checklist to help you evaluate your physical plant:

A. Facility Exterior

■ Access in and out of parking lot.
■ Access for handicapped.
■ Attractiveness of building exterior.
■ Access into building.
■ Signs to indicate your office.

B. Reception Area

■ Easy access through doorways.
■ Pleasing colors, attractive decor.
■ Proper lighting, not too bright, especially for elderly.
■ Comfort and utility of furniture.
■ Special children's area, where needed.
■ Interesting magazines, even videotapes.
■ Cleanliness.

C. Examination Rooms

■ Bright and cheerful decor.
■ Appropriate drapes.
■ Reading material.
■ Climate control.
■ Comfortable exam tables.

From the moment patients arrive, they ought to sense an inviting, professional practice that takes pride in caring for their comfort and convenience.

Your Staff. How many physicians really pay attention to the attitudes of their staffs? Yet your patients' experiences with your employees are a big part of the impressions they form of your total product. For example:

On her last office visit, Ms. Jones had her blood pressure taken because she was concerned about having hypertension. But when she asked the nurse what the recording was, she got a curt: "The doctor will tell you."

Figure 9-B
POINTS OF PATIENTS' PERCEPTIONS

- Call for Appointment
- Arrival for Appointment
- Reception Area
- Treatment by Staff
- Interaction With Physician
- After-visit contact

That's what the nurse said. What Ms. Jones heard, however, was, "I'm too busy. Don't bother me. You have to wait for the doctor. Now sit down, and be quiet." The nurse could have handled the inquiry far more tactfully and easily. All she had to do was smile and say, "The doctor will be with you very shortly. As you know he's very precise, so he likes to answer such questions himself."

If patients feel your people are friendly and helpful, they're already thinking in terms of a good, overall experience. But if they feel the staff is hurried and too busy for them, their experience starts—or ends—on a sour note.

Many practices have had marketing problems solely because of the staffs. Businesses have long recognized the importance of employees' attitudes, and many hold regular training sessions on customer relations. American Telephone and Telegraph Company employees now end each phone conversation with customers by saying, "Thank you for calling A.T.&T." We all know this has happened since deregulation and the attendant increase in competition.

One physician asked us how in the world he could evaluate the attitude of his staff unless he got specific complaints? One way would be to take the initiative and ask patients about specific employees. You can do that through a patient survey or direct conversation. The need for feedback is particularly appropriate with new patients, who haven't established relationships with employees, and who therefore may be willing to give unbiased opinions.

Sometimes, faithful patients won't complain about your staff because they like you and don't want to hurt your feelings. While they may not leave your practice because of your staff, it's doubtful that they'll refer other people to you.

Ask patients several quick questions to get some idea of how your staff is viewed. Two examples:

"Did Ms. Smith check your weight and blood pressure?"

That gives the patient a chance to discuss the encounter and let you know how well Ms. Smith is doing her job of pleasing patients.

"You know, Mr. Green, I think my staff is having a bad day."

That's a good leading question and will inspire the more timid patients to speak up. After all, if the doctor feels his staff is having an off day, then the patients may gather the courage to corroborate it, and complaints may flow. On the other hand, you may find them defending your employees, which would be good news, indeed.

Your office personnel are a reflection of you. They should bolster the total image of your practice. They, as well as you, should always remember what business you are in. One doctor we know has put up a plaque in his office that reads, "We are in the business of making patients healthy and happy."

Your Attitude. Physicians tend to spend most of their time diagnosing and treating, and little time honing their interpersonal skills. Yet those skills can significantly influence the patient's total experience in your office.

Far too many physicians spend too much time worrying about how *many* patients they see, and not enough time worrying about *how* they see them. Yes, to be financially successful you have to pay attention to the bottom line; the total number of patients is important. But the bottom line doesn't always indicate the long-term success of a practice. In fact, it may be the very thing that's adding up to patients' adverse attitudes. Seeing too many patients today may result in seeing too few a year from now.

The basic problem is that many doctors are unwilling or unable to communicate. They try to reach their patients when discussing medicine, but don't really respond to the patient's basic desire for empathy, undivided attention, and understanding of their entire problem. That may involve many factors outside the field of medicine. What about a recent divorce, chronically ill parents, a lost job?

To communicate, according to Webster's dictionary, is to "interchange thoughts." But an interchange takes two parties. You aren't really communicating with patients when interviews consist entirely of you expressing opinions or giving information, or when you ask only for medical histories and descriptions of symptoms. The reasons for illness, or the repercussions from illness, often extend far beyond the boundaries of traditional medicine.

No, we're not trying to turn all physicians into psychiatrists. Not really. But every doctor will have to learn to function to some extent in terms of the psychological needs of his or her patients.

We can't stress too often that one of the major pitfalls is not properly assessing what patients really mean when they complain that you're not spending enough time with them. They're not talking about how far the hands of the clock moved. They're talking about the *quality* of the time: how attentive you were.

They want you to at least give the *impression* of not being hurried, of not racing quickly through the evaluation to get to the next patient. Patients should leave your examining room feeling that while you were with them, they were your *only* concern. That's often harder to accomplish than to diagnose the condition and prescribe the treatment. But if you don't treat patients' perceptions of you, along with their medical problems, you're lowering the value of your services in their eyes.

Keep in mind, too, that your patients' perceptions of your practice may also be affected, positively or negatively, by any follow-up contact from you or your staff after they leave your office. *(See Fig. 9-C)*

THE QUALITY
OF YOUR PRODUCT

Throughout this chapter we've discussed wants, needs, and perceptions. The real bottom line, however, is that the clinical product you deliver must be of the highest quality. Otherwise, all your other marketing efforts might as well be junked.

True enough, you can take a substandard product, put a lot of hoopla behind it, and market it to almost anyone. But if the product doesn't satisfy the consumer, it will eventually fail, no matter how well it's promoted. Remember the Edsel automobile produced by Ford in the late 1950s? Millions of dollars were spent on a well-conceived advertising plan. The trouble was, the public didn't want the Edsel. Not that it was a bad automobile. It just didn't satisfy the needs of the public.

Your health-care product is no different. Physicians must provide a quality product that meets the expectations of a sophisticated public, and the standards of the world's greatest health-care system. Make no mistake, most of today's consumers can tell the difference between poor medicine and quality care. They may be fooled in your reception area, but once they've received your complete care, they have a pretty accurate idea of your worth. They can differentiate between a quality physician and one "just trying to get rich."

PUT YOURSELF IN
YOUR PATIENTS' SHOES

Product quality, and the patient's perception of it, is especially important when you're considering the introduction of a new product. That's when you especially need to put yourself in the shoes of potential users.

Take the case of an orthopedist friend in the Southwest, who wanted to increase the number of younger, athletically oriented patients in his practice. Since he was a jogging and fitness enthusiast, it was easy for him to evolve a sports medicine thrust to his practice. He attended special sports seminars and visited extensively with his athletic, non-physician friends. He even had his nurse read up on the subject. In conjunction with offering sports medicine as an extra service, he became more involved with sports teams and a jogging association. As a result, his sports practice boomed.

HOW TO DEVELOP
PRODUCT STRATEGIES

For each marketing goal, there must be a marketing plan. And the way to plan is to view each goal in the light of your market segment priorities, and the marketing mix to be applied.

The best way to gain insight into the development of product strategies is to take case studies and show how the problems were dealt with from the product aspect.

The Case of the Disappearing Patients

An internist in a small urban community became worried about a decline in her patient load. She was also aware of a recent influx of new physicians into the community.

Data. As part of her initial marketing evaluation, she gathered this representative marketing research data:

- The average decline in patient load was 5 per week.
- An appreciable number of her exiting patients were joining alternative-delivery systems.
- Of surveyed patients, 65 percent complained about difficulty in dealing with her office staff.
- Of female patients, 75 percent went to other physicians for routine gynecological care.
- Of those women, 80 percent would have preferred to receive that care from her, if it were available.

Goals. The next step was to develop specific marketing goals to stem the tide of dropouts. Here are the three goals she set:

1. Evaluate the effectiveness of the staff and refine their interpersonal skills.
2. Evaluate current gynecological procedures and offer a revised service.
3. Find out what other reasons patients have for leaving in favor of alternative-delivery systems.

Product Strategies. After data had been collected, practice problems identified, and marketing goals established, she developed strategies to achieve each goal. She then had to choose her marketing mix. For our purposes, we'll review only the planning that involved the first P—the Product. Here are her strategies:

Goal 1: Improve staff effectiveness.
Strategies:
- Hold meetings to involve the staff in shaping the overall goals for the practice.
- Help each staff member improve interpersonal skills, and explain the effect each person's behavior has on the success of the practice.

Goal 2: Investigate gynecological care.
Strategies:
- Evaluate current expertise in providing this service.
- Attend various courses on office gynecology and strengthen skills in examinations.

Goal 3: Determine why patients leave the practice.
Strategies:
- Use an exit questionnaire to find out why patients leave.
- Pinpoint their reasons for leaving, and re-evaluate strategies in the light of those findings.

The Case of the Contact Lenses

An ophthalmologist in a highly competitive city needed to find ways to attract a larger patient base. This physician had an interest and an expertise in contact lenses.

Data. His market research revealed the following:

- The surrounding area is highly competitive, with several nonphysician facilities offering contact-lens care.
- Of his current patients, 55 percent wear contacts.
- Of those, 80 percent desire to receive total contact-lens care from the practice.
- A large number of potential patients are current, or possibly future, contact-lens wearers.

Goals. These three marketing goals resulted:
1. Find the strengths and weaknesses of the competition.
2. Provide total contact-lens care, including evaluation, manufacture, and fitting, for current and potential patients.
3. Market this service as a source of generating potential patients and retaining current ones.

Product Strategies. The following strategies were then chosen to meet the goals.

Goal 1: Discover weaknesses in the competition.
Strategies:
- Devise a method of listing each competitor with strengths and weaknesses.
- Evaluate current product in the light of weaknesses found in competitors' operations. These weak points can then become target market areas.

Figure 9-C
MEDICAL SERVICE DELIVERY

Patient/Practice Need	Marketing Strategy
Convenience	Flexible Hours
Less Waiting Time	Better Scheduling
More Information	Educational Material
More Time With Doctor	Spend More Quality Time
Specific Services	Evaluate Scope of Services
Cooperative Staff	Develop New Services
	Staff Involvement/Education

Goal 2: Offer total contact-lens care.
Strategy: Broaden and upgrade the current product to make sure it meets the express needs of both current and potential patients.

Goal 3: Strengthen product and service.
Strategy: Review the current product and fine-tune the approach to the service so that the strengths equal those of the competition, and the weaknesses are eliminated or reduced.

Summary

Those are a few examples of how the physician's product enters into overall marketing planning. In this chapter we've considered only the concept of Product and its influence. In the next chapter we'll take up Price, often the most important part of marketing.

Reference

1. Gwinner RF, Brown SW: *Marketing: An Environmental Perspective.* St. Paul, MN: West Publishing Co., 1977.

CHAPTER 10

Creating fair and flexible fees

"Would you look at this bill I got from my doctor!"

Who hasn't heard those familiar words? Whether the bill was justified makes no difference. The fact that consumers—both employers and patients—see the cost of health care as too high creates many of the competitive problems facing traditional medicine today. And that brings us to the second component P of your marketing mix: Price.

During a conversation at a recent business luncheon, a physician friend made the mistake of saying that patients weren't concerned with cost so long as they got quality care. Several of his friends, who represented different businesses, responded quickly. They said patients were indeed concerned, because many businesses were demanding a greater investment by the employee in the costs of health care. They added that physicians who don't recognize the importance of cost just might find their patients going elsewhere.

The reasons for escalating medical costs are arguable; the indisputable fact is that patients are paying considerably more for health care today than they did just a few years ago. It's important for physicians to appreciate the effect their prices will have on their current and future practice.

The issue of pricing has generally been avoided by the medical profession. Fee-for-service physicians have, for the most part, charged what they wanted. Few patients resisted because their insurance coverage insulated them from the true costs of their care. The typical physician still enters practice and either charges what his or her new partners charge, or asks around and matches the going rate for the community. But the environment may no longer be right for such a pricing system.

PRICING RIGHT
Like your product, your price is an indicator of the quality of your services, and it's used by patients in their overall evaluation of your practice. It may not be the most obvious element, but in today's economy it's one of the most important, and it can become either a powerful marketing asset, or a devastating liability.

Many believe pricing will quickly become the most important element of your entire marketing mix. Why? Because of the escalating costs of health care and the emergence of a more active role by business and third-party payers in determining the ultimate price.

As business has been forced to pay higher and higher employee health benefits, its role in the decision-making process continues to expand. When you consider that a higher percentage of the cost of a new automobile is due to employee health benefits than to the cost of steel, you can quickly see why business has become concerned about health costs.

Patients are also assuming a more active role, both by taking on greater financial responsibility, and by becoming highly sophisticated in shopping for health care. The rapid escalation of enrollment in HMOs and other types of health plans is testimony to the patients' willingness to accept alternative systems based on cost. So to survive in this increasingly price-sensitive environment, you must develop a better understanding of marketing principles that relate to pricing, and how they can be used to your advantage.

Now, none of this should be construed as a drive for doctors to automatically reduce fees, although external pressures are working to do just that. The marketing discipline doesn't advocate high or low prices. As a matter of fact, there are successful high- and low-priced marketers in almost all areas of the business world. Example: Premium ice creams are on the high end of one market, H. & R. Block on the low end of another.

Though much of this chapter concerns the pressure to lower fees, the fact remains that a physician who is perceived as providing extraordinary care, skills, and services will be able to maintain fees higher than most other physicians.

PRICING OBJECTIVES

In a classic article in the *American Economic Review*, "Pricing Objectives in Large Companies,"[1] Robert F. Lanzillotti found in his comprehensive research that large, successful corporations achieved four main goals. Not all apply to physicians, but they can help you make pricing decisions.

Target Return

Many corporations base their pricing on the return they wish to make on their investment or sales. The cost of delivering the service is calculated by considering overhead, taxes, and other expenses. The price to the consumer is then set at the desired percentage above that cost. If the corporation desires a 10 percent profit margin, then the cost to the consumer will be 10 percent above the cost of delivering the service.

Physicians have generally been considered poor business people. This is certainly not always the case, but in many instances, doctors don't conduct their practices primarily as businesses. How many even think of their profession as delivering a product? How many even know how much it costs them to deliver a particular product? If they knew, pricing would be less of a problem. To ensure profitability, they could simply set the price of a product or service at a particular level above its actual cost.

During a marketing consultation, we asked a large group of physicians how the business aspects of their practices were run.

"We run a potentially profitable business like a five-and-dime store," one physician responded. "We simply don't know how much to charge because we don't know how much it costs to deliver."

This honest appraisal illustrates how many marketing problems are caused by the failure to understand basic economic principles.

Market Share

Many companies use price aggressively to maintain or improve their share of a certain market. They price their product or service to secure a preset market share. If they achieve or improve that share, then pricing was successful. If their market share falls off, they re-evaluate overall pricing policies.

Of the various approaches to pricing, this one could be the most detrimental to physicians. If you were to wait for your share of the market to decline before you re-evaluate pricing, it might be too late. Pricing strategies must be reviewed *before* your share of the market is lost. Nevertheless, the idea of market share and its relation to pricing is becoming increasingly relevant for today's physician.

Price Stability

In many industries, the message is: Don't rock the boat. Rather than declare a price war, sellers match their competitors' prices. That way, one can't get a bigger share of the market by undercutting the others.

It's almost an unspoken law that major-brand distributors all set prices at about the same level. The effects of moving away from a "price-stable system" can be remembered from the days of the gas price war. When one major company lowered its prices dramatically, the others had to follow, and the battle was on. Today, we see these effects in the deregulated airline industry.

Does the objective sound familiar? It should. The vast majority of practices put values on their services and products based on the principle of price stability. Physicians have traditionally been afraid to go against the mainstream in establishing fees. So what's happened? Alternative systems, unafraid to break with traditional pricing, have moved in and cut deeply into fee-for-service practices.

Meeting Competition

"We will match any price our competitors offer!" is a common ploy of businesses to price their product or service at whatever level is necessary to compete. Some industries will offer their services and products at such low costs that potential competitors don't even bother to challenge them. Then, once the market is assured, the price can be raised gradually to profitable levels.

Many of the alternative health-care systems use this approach. It often works because the hardest part is to attract patients to a new service. Once they're enrolled, many become satisfied and are reluctant to change again, even though the price may eventually rise to what their original physicians charged.

THE PATIENT'S VIEW OF PRICE

Patients increasingly believe they should participate in decisions about the cost of their medical care. They're assuming a greater role in decisions about testing, prescriptions, hospitals, and even specific modes of care—all based on cost.

Patients will bear an even greater financial risk in obtaining health care in the future as employers and third-party carriers encourage, or demand, utilization of cost-effective hospitals and physicians. In many states, traditional third-party carriers—such as "the Blues"— require patients to use preferred providers. If you're not one of these providers, your patients covered under Blue Cross and Blue Shield will have a very tough decision to make. For physicians to keep these patients without becoming "discount doctors," they must look to marketing for innovative approaches to the problems of pricing. To use pricing as an effective marketing tool, look at how patients perceive the cost of your product.

THE CHANGING FACE OF INSURANCE

Payment for health care was once very easy. For the most part, patients didn't have to worry about paying the bills. They bought health insurance. Patients would go to the doctor with this attitude: "Do whatever you want, and do it the best way you can. Price is no object; my insurance will pay it."

Probably, at one time, patients were more worried about quality and less about who paid the bills, but not now. While it's true that most people have insurance to cover their medical bills, carriers are recouping the higher cost of medical benefits by charging higher premiums, requiring higher copayments, and directing patients to preferred and lower-cost providers. Patients are reacting to these higher premiums by either limiting their coverage to major medical policies or, in the case of many elderly people, simply dropping everything but their Medicare. The steady decline in outpatient visits can, in part, be attributed to patients simply not being able to utilize services as they once could, because of cost.

Corporations, which buy 80 to 85 percent of all health insurance, are concerned because coverage is an increasingly expensive employee benefit. These companies used to give their employees a choice of where to receive their care. Now, they seek high-quality, low-priced alternatives, and demand that their employees patronize those facilities. But how can a company dictate where its employees spend their health-care dollars?

Other than closed-staff HMOs, no policy denies clients the right to use the physician of their choice. However, many insurance companies are seeking innovative ways to "suggest" better avenues of care. Foote, Cone & Belding, an advertising firm with 2,500 employees, used to cover 100 percent of most hospital costs, and 80 percent of doctor bills. But when faced with the rising costs of maintaining that coverage, they rewrote the policy.

Under the new policy, only 80 percent of hospital charges are covered, but complete coverage is provided for a variety of nonhospital treatments. The insurance will still pick up 80 percent of a surgeon's bill, but only when a second opinion verifies the need. Otherwise, payment is 50 percent. You can begin to see how freedom of choice is being limited by these changes, which can't help but affect your practice and how patients perceive the cost of your product.

You may think that this sort of thing really only affects hospital care, and not your office practice. Not true. Blue Cross and Blue Shield in Atlanta and other cities recently proposed a system-wide PPO. They will provide maximum coverage only for those policy holders who go to designated physicians and hospitals. In return for guaranteed patient referrals, the physicians and hospitals agree to discount prices. The idea has spread to many other insurance carriers.

"I'm not signing up," responded an angry physician. "My patients will stay with me rather than go to a discount doctor they don't know." Maybe so. Probably not.

Perhaps the only force stronger than established patient loyalty is patient economics. And the price of health care and insurance coverage are powerful deterrents to established physician loyalty. Couple those with the changing attitudes in employer coverage, and you have adequate reasons for many families to leave their lifelong physicians. You can ignore the facts, but many patients simply can't afford to pay the difference between your bill and what their insurance will cover. Ultimately, they'll stop coming to you.

During a recent practice consultation for some internists, several exit surveys were taken. The internists were astonished to find that many patients who had grown up in the practice were leaving because their insurance would cover only an HMO or a PPO physician. The patients were embarrassed and saddened, but the economic pressure outweighed their loyalty. Not all patients will leave, but many will have no choice.

The internists then asked if this meant they should become members of a prepaid group. From a marketing viewpoint, that's a tough question. Several years ago the decision to join was primarily a philosophical one. Today, such formerly contemplative considerations are almost totally concerned with economics alone.

Our internists group doesn't have to join a prepaid or discounted practice to survive. But if they cling to the idea that patients will continue to pay whatever they're charged, they'll eventually find themselves out of business. Not even the strongest practice will be able to get away with that.

Are there any health-care providers who don't believe that the policy of Diagnosis Related Grouping (DRG) won't eventually make its way into doctors' offices? As we write this, proposals are being submitted from powerful sources to expand the scope of the DRG program. Mandatory assignment of Medicare patients, as well as a prohibition against charging the patient the difference between your fee and the insurance payment are also looming up before us. The important point is that physicians must begin to look at pricing from a marketing perspective. Later in this chapter we'll discuss specific marketing strategies that can help in this rapidly changing, price-conscious environment.

THE REAL COST
OF YOUR CARE

Physicians rarely know exactly how much it costs to provide a service, so the pricing of each service is usually based on what everyone else charges. In most cases this approach works, because all physicians within a given economic area charge basically the same. But is it good marketing?

The amount you bill for a given service should be based on sound economics. Physicians can't attend a seminar or read a book to learn about pricing, because charges must be tailored to the current cost of delivering the particular service, the overhead, and the profit margin of the practice.

Physicians must continue to remind themselves that patients are paying for their service in one way or another. They're paying higher premiums for the privilege of that coverage, and they're paying a greater differential cost between what you charge and what their insurance pays.

Strategic marketing suggests that the best guideline is to price services so they are beneficial to the majority of patients within the practice. Marketing principles, however, suggest that if a service is too highly priced, the marketplace will quickly let you know simply by not patronizing the practice.

Does that mean you must charge less in order to attract more patients? No, but it does mean you should charge only what the market—or your priority market segments—will bear. It also means that patients must be kept informed of what your charges are, and that you must keep in touch with how they respond to the charges. You must be willing not only to discuss fees openly, but to solicit patient reactions.

How can you market your fees? By making patients aware of both the quality of the service and the cost of delivering it. Make sure they're aware that the price of an office visit includes not only the visit itself, but easy access to you by phone, availability at night and on weekends, and comprehensive quality care. You'll have a marketing problem if your charges are high and your services aren't perceived to be readily accessible or comprehensive.

Consumer's Perception:
Expect It to Be Expensive _____ The emergence of a free marketplace for medical care exposes physicians to another business axiom. A consumer's *perception* of cost is many times more important than the *price* itself. Think about that for a moment. Patients have a perception that the price of the service is going to be high even before they know the cost. Consumers have been preconditioned to expect medical care to be expensive. When told that America is spending a billion dollars a day on health care, many will try to figure out how much of that bill is theirs. If prices aren't openly discussed from the beginning, you can hardly blame them for resisting.

Consider the last restaurant you went to that didn't list the prices on the menu. Most of us in that situation would reach for our wallets to make sure we'd brought credit cards. We'd assume the prices were high. Why else would they not display the cost to their customers? Other than in such a restaurant, where else does high-price anxiety exist? *(See Fig. 10-A)*

Don't look too far, because the same principle applies to physicians who don't want to discuss fees. And if you don't, your patients' apprehensions will be automatically aroused.

Nonmonetary Cost _____ Many times patients pay a high price for a product that can't be measured in dollars and cents. Not many physicians realize the fear patients may have when they go to the doctor. This fear can put a heavy toll on them and their families. We're not talking about the fear of pain, but the fear of the unknown—that something might be seriously wrong, and that whatever is wrong might severely affect their jobs, family lives, or economic situations.

That fear must be dealt with by an empathetic and compassionate physician. Otherwise, the patient might decide that the emotional price is too high to pay, and simply not return to the practice. Physicians must openly discuss any fears patients might have, and be pre-

Figure 10-A
EASING THE COST OF CARE

Patient Concern	Physician Can
Price of Care	Revise Fee Structure
Payment	Vary Billing
Insurance	Maximize Reimbursement Options
Lost Wages	Offer Flexible Hours

Figure 10-B
LOWERING NON-MONETARY COSTS

To Reduce Patients'	Physician Can
Fear	Give Reassurance
Apprehension	Acknowledge and Talk About It
Waiting Time	Adjust Scheduling

pared to help them cope. That's not just good marketing; it's quality medicine. *(See Fig. 10-B)*

On the more practical side, physicians must appreciate the *inconvenience* created by a trip to the doctor. A physician friend was recently discussing an appointment with his accountant. He was worried that the accountant wouldn't be able to see him after hours.

"Why do you think he should wait and see you?"

"Because, if I go during the day, I lose too much patient time."

The first impression was that this doctor was concerned about losing time with his patients, but the more he talked, the more it became apparent that he was concerned about losing *money*.

Are your patients really any different? In order to come to your office, most of them are leaving their work, taking sick leave, or missing business appointments that may result in lost income or bad vibes from the boss.

Physicians must be as appreciative of patients' time as they are of their own. Marketing techniques should be developed to assure a minimum of waiting and inconvenience. As we'll discuss in the next chapter, the more convenient and less time consuming your patients perceive your services to be, the more they'll use them, and the less concerned they'll be about the price. A patient who spends wasted time in your reception area will think of your price as higher than it actually is, simply because he or she begins to figure lost wages into the total cost.

PRICING STRATEGIES
The question remains: "How can you use pricing as a positive marketing tool?" Let's take some marketing problems that deal with pricing and discuss specific strategies. Assume that a practice has collected the appropriate market research data and has identified three problems. The patients:

■ Perceive the cost of the service as too high.
■ Are unaware of the pricing within the practice.
■ Want help in paying their bills.

A physician in such a practice might begin marketing planning to meet those problems with these strategies:

Problem 1:
The Price Isn't Right

Goal 1: Evaluate cost of services.
Strategies:

- Utilize standard economic techniques to determine actual cost of each service offered by the practice.
- Gather information on comparative pricing within the community.
- Establish an appropriate profit margin based on realistic expectations and anticipated inflation changes.

Before you can gain control of your pricing and its effect on patients, you must accurately establish what it costs to provide a particular service. How can you discuss the price of an X-ray with a patient without first knowing how much it will cost you? Discussions based solely on the position, "That's what others are charging," will quickly become defensive and counterproductive. Patients are much more receptive to sound economic reasons than they are to rhetoric.

Competitive pricing may seem offensive, yet physicians should consider adjusting their prices so they're more highly competitive. Some physicians, such as surgeons, whose services are primarily covered by third-party payers, must also look at the effect their pricing will have on their being included or excluded by certain carriers.

Goal 2: Price services effectively, taking into account facts obtained in Goal 1 and the effect pricing will have on patient population.
Strategies:

- Review market research data and develop an economic profile of the practice.
- Develop an idea of how many patients are covered by insurance, and profile experience you've had with reimbursement in the past.

Many physicians, especially newer ones, fail to take their patients' economic situation into consideration. That doesn't mean you must charge the minimum your patients can afford. It does mean, however, that your approach should be tailored to their economic condition.

A strong case can be made for scaling prices in certain situations. Many practices will either adjust or waive fees in unusual cases. The overall effect on your practice can be quite positive. It's good public relations. Other patients, both current and future, will hear how you helped a patient who was temporarily laid off. They'll also hear if you refused to help.

Problem 2:
The Price Is Unknown

Goal: Inform patients of prices.
Strategies:
- Distribute to all patients a practice brochure explaining prices and business policies.
- Publish similar information in a practice newsletter.
- Ask patients at the end of visits if they have any questions regarding the bill.
- Educate office staff on the importance of explaining charges.
- Have receptionist or office manager ask, when patients check out, if they have any questions about the charges.
- Post a sign in the office encouraging patients to ask about charges.
- Obtain sampling of patients having problems with their bills to see if any relate to confusion about charges.

Physicians must make every attempt to communicate individually with patients regarding fees. The more openness you have regarding your pricing, the less confusion and resentment there will be.

Problem 3:
Patients Need Help to Pay

Goal: Help patients find the means to pay their bills.
Strategies:
- Develop, or refine, sound business policies for the office.
- Make sure all patients are aware of those policies.
- Help with insurance evaluation so patients can learn beforehand what their insurance companies will pay for a potential service; this applies especially to elective procedures, such as plastic surgery.
- Help with insurance forms and update current bill into a "super-bill" summarizing all services rendered.
- Offer innovative credit options in special cases.
- Consider accepting credit cards.

Several years ago, physicians felt they didn't have the responsibility for mediating between the patient and the insurance company. Many still feel that way. Today's environment, however, requires that physicians reconsider their role. Patients need an advocate in the confusing maze of insurance. If the physician's office assumes some of the advocate role, patients will be less likely to change to prepaid coverage plans.

Your practice must consider helping patients answer questions on coverage, filling out and filing forms, and acting as a patient advocate with third-party payers. The attitude that your "contract" is with the patient rather than the insurance company is understandable. But in today's competitive environment, that attitude can be detrimental. No one suggests that you have to do everything for patients, but whatever help you can give will be interpreted as a positive signal that you're on their side.

Those are only three of many pricing strategies that can be incorporated into a marketing plan. A number of others can apply to specific situations. Four examples:

Situation 1:
Make the Most of Medicare

Goal: Get Medicare reimbursement for eligible patients.
Strategies:
- Make sure patients understand their "coinsurance" responsibilities.
- Accept assignments to secure a continuing patient base of Medicare recipients.
- Analyze trends in home health-care coverage and devise strategies to incorporate them into the practice's services.
- Discount the difference between Medicare coverage and the patient's balance of the bill.

Situation 2:
Attract Industrial Patients

Goal: Provide a practice that will appeal to industries and make them willing to send you patients.
Strategies:
- Discount your charges to a specific industrial plant in exchange for workers' compensation patients.
- Offer a package deal on pre-employment physicals. A flat rate of $50 for a $75 physical won't hurt the practice much. Physicals could be done at one time to decrease your cost, and could provide incentive for the company to give you more business.

Situation 3:
Speed Collection, Lower Cost

Goal: Collect payment at the time of service.
Strategies:
- Reduce bill by a few dollars if paid at time of service.
- Request payment at time of service; tell patients through newsletter or brochure how prompt payment reduces long-term costs to them and you.

Situation 4:
Potential Patients Fear Cost

Goal: Attract patients by reducing their fear of unaffordable costs.
Strategy: Offer new patients free interviews to provide opportunity to discuss services, prices, and financial strategies of your practice.

Summary
The cost of your services may be one of the most powerful deterrents to people seeking your care. But if you incorporate effective pricing strategies and communication, your price will work for you, not against you.

Reference

1. Lanzillotti RF: Pricing objectives in large companies. *American Economic Review*, December 1958, 921-940.

CHAPTER 11

You've got to be accessible

Most, if not all, of the alternative health-care delivery systems competing with private practitioners have succeeded on the assumption that traditional medicine doesn't bother to satisfy the needs of a convenience-oriented society. Nowhere does this hold more true than in the Place component of the marketing mix. This is in the area of accessibility—the times and places when you're available to your patients.

So long as the patients were out there, literally "waiting" in filled-up waiting rooms, doctors had no problems about availability. Doctors just took patients when they could get to them.

No longer are "patients" crowding in like sheep, willing to put up with discomfort and inconvenience. Why should they? They don't have to when they buy clothes, food, or banking services. Why should they be compelled to wait unnaturally long periods of time for medical attention? As a result, the competitive environment is taking a fearful toll from doctors who stubbornly keep practicing in a primitive manner.

BEING THERE

Your customer is the one who ultimately determines the right times and the right places for you to be. The success of McDonald's as a fast-food restaurant chain is an excellent example of that.

McDonald's built its operation around giving the customers food where and when they wanted it. This meant being located close to major traffic arteries, providing food quickly, and expanding the hours of operation.

Unless you're a diehard who stubbornly clings to the antiquated ideas that (a) "patients" are not "customers," (b) they're not buying anything/you're not selling anything, and (c) the whole relationship takes place in some never-never land, free of the laws of commerce, you must now appreciate the necessity of being convenient to your customers. Of course, if you do stick with an outworn image of a doctor's place in the world, some patients may continue to come to you when they have a special problem, or a long "shopping list" of problems. On that basis, you may survive, but you won't prosper. And you won't be serving your patients to the extent that you could.

GETTING TO CUSTOMERS
AND VICE VERSA

In marketing terms, distribution is the process of bringing services to consumers. In traditional business, distribution of a product involves manufacturer, wholesaler, retailer, and finally consumer. A similar analogy exists in medicine. *(Fig. 11-A)*

In their *Health Care Marketing Plans*, Stephen Hillestad and Eric Berkowitz describe direct and indirect distribution systems.[1] Here's how those systems and an agent-included network function.

Figure 11-A
HEALTH-CARE DISTRIBUTION

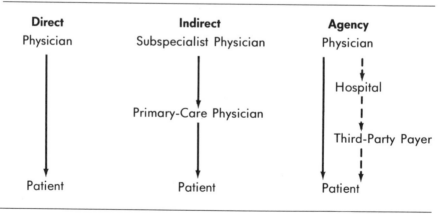

Direct Delivery —————————————— A direct system, or channel, exists when the provider of the health-care service deals directly with the consumer. Primary-care physicians are part of this, delivering services directly to their patients, and relying primarily on themselves to generate new patients.

Indirect Delivery —————————————— Physicians, hospitals, and third-party payers are the leading characters in providing the distribution of health-care services. Hospitals, through their emergency rooms and other programs, refer patients to members of their medical staffs. Further, they provide the setting for much of the sophisticated care provided. Like physicians, hospitals are now feeling the pressures of our changing environment. As a result, many of these institutions are using marketing to help them cope.

Third-party payers also influence the distribution of health care. Though they don't provide a physical location for that process, their encouragement of second opinions stimulates patients to go to more physicians. Also, the moves of government and private insurers to shorten hospital stays have helped to develop the home health-care industry.

Why is it important to recognize the different channels of distribution? Because marketing efforts will vary, depending upon whether there is someone between you and your potential patients.

Primary-care physicians must concentrate their marketing efforts directly on the patients. Referral-dependent physicians must concentrate on the physicians who play the roles of agents, who initiate contacts with the patients. But to retain the customers they get, referral-dependent doctors must be sure to orient their practices to their patients as well.

Though these channels of distribution have always been defined fairly well, many doctors are now bypassing referral physicians, and are marketing directly to the consumers. Practitioners of plastic surgery, for example, are providing free information, lectures, and media programs to educate the public about the benefits of their specialty. Traditionally thought of as being in an indirect channel, these physicians are bypassing their referring doctors and are going directly to consumers. While this can result in effective marketing, it poses a threat to primary-care physicians.

Another innovative marketing strategy that bypasses traditional channels is a joint venture among indirect-channel physicians and hospitals. Hospitals take the place of the referring physicians, marketing particular services by referring the potential patient to a specialist who delivers the service.

A hospital in Georgia marketed its facility through a campaign focused on the benefits of cosmetic surgery. When a patient inquired about the services, he or she was referred to one of the plastic surgeons on staff. The campaign was highly successful—thousands of calls were received. The hospital benefited from a large inpatient census, and the plastic surgeons got more patients. But many primary-care specialists felt the threat from this positioning of a third party between the patient and the ultimate provider.

To some observers of the changing medical scene, this "interference" by hospitals and third-party payers is contributing to the rising costs of health care, and may mean that primary-care physicians will no longer be the "gatekeepers" of the medical distribution system.

DISTRIBUTION TRENDS

It's important for you to appreciate some of the recent distribution trends being used by competing services to satisfy specific needs. In gaining an understanding of why these trends work, you'll be better able to plot your own strategies to counter them.

Convenient Positioning

"Storefront" clinics are springing up all over the country because those who run them realize the convenience they offer by positioning themselves in high-traffic areas—the shopping mall being the most obvious example. In major malls you now find primary-care centers, diagnostic clinics, and high blood pressure clinics, to name a few. These "shops" are cleverly drawing their customers from the ready-made potential patient pool of people attracted to the mall by the promotions and advertisements of the commercial establishments.

"But if people come to the mall to shop, what makes you think they'll spend time waiting to see a doctor?" asked one physician.

Well, for one thing, they don't have to spend time waiting. Patients checking in at many storefront clinics are given beepers—that's right, the good old standby of the busy physician. They can then go about their shopping; when the doctor is ready to see them, they get a beep. So what are the storefront clinics selling? Convenience. And the public loves it.

Often, the strategic location of a facility can be as important as its convenience. Traditional business philosophy has always followed the edict that if you can get the customers into the store, chances are pretty good they'll buy something. Sears utilizes this idea effectively by locating many of its stores at the entrances of large shopping malls. The plan is to have as many people as possible walk through Sears to get to the rest of the mall— because when they walk through, many will stop and buy.

Knowing that people need convenient professional services, Sears has added financial and real estate counseling, insurance and dental services. Consumers can now get their teeth cleaned, filled, or replaced while shopping at Sears. And often, they can do it without even making appointments. They can check up on their health and buy a garden hose in the same place. Some large-scale retailers also may add medical services to their list of conveniences for the consumer.

Convenient Hours

Patients are not always comfortable with the 9 to 5 hours offered by most physicians. They prefer doctors who are ready to accommodate themselves to the patients' schedules. Alternative delivery systems, therefore, are often open earlier in the morning, later in the day, and on weekends.

Though it's most effective, this system has weaknesses, such as non-availability in the middle of the night. Yet many patients don't seem overly concerned about lack of coverage from late evening to 8 a.m. Many feel they can call their "regular" doctor or, if necessary, go to a hospital emergency room.

Even if a doctor's office hours are convenient, "waiting time" can become a problem to patients. This form of inconvenience includes the hours, days, or weeks that it may take to see a physician once a patient requests an appointment, and the time it takes in minutes or hours for the patient to see the doctor once he or she is in the office. Offices that require a new patient to wait weeks for an appointment are already establishing in the patient's mind a restless feeling of inconvenience.

Recognizing the importance of first impressions, one doctor we know has arranged her schedule so she can see new patients within three days of their calls—or the same day, if need be.

In-office waits are often unavoidable, but they represent a major source of patient irritation. Consumer-sensitive practices are going out of their way to phone patients when appointments have to be delayed, and to tell them upon arrival at the office the reasons for the delays.

Convenient positioning and convenient hours are key accessibility strategies now in use. If you understand why and how they are used, it will be easier for you to develop your own accessibility and distribution strategies. *(See Fig. 11-B)*

Figure 11-B
ACCESSIBILITY STRATEGIES

Patient Need	Marketing Strategy
Better Parking	Offer Free Parking
	Join Private Lot
	Improve Lighting
Convenient Public Transportation	Publish Bus Schedules
Home Care	Arrange Transportation
	Offer Home Health Care
Convenient Location	Study Feasibility of Satellite Location and Office Sharing
Convenient Time	Evaluate Scheduling
	Stagger Office Hours
	Extend Office Hours

ACCESSIBILITY STRATEGIES

If you have a quality *product*, offered at the right *price*, good marketing dictates that to be effective you must offer your product in the right *place*. When referring to a medical service, place generally means both accessibility and availability—that is, not only the right place but also the right time.

Let's look at some specific strategies you can use in solving a variety of marketing problems related to accessibility and availability. Assume you've identified four problems of accessibility that you want to solve. Here's how to go about it:

Problem 1:
Inconvenient Access

Goal: Find out why patients see your services as inconvenient.

Strategies: Conduct a patient survey to identify specific causes of dissatisfaction. Your location may not be the reason patients find your practice inconvenient. A number of other factors may come to light. For example:

■ *Poor parking.* Evaluate existing parking for: number of spaces needed vs. spaces available; expense; lighting (especially if you have night hours); and security (especially if your practice is in a heavily populated area). If your parking is expensive or unsafe, make arrangements with a nearby garage or lot for free, well-lighted, secure parking for each patient for at least two hours.

- *Poor access.* Make sure there are adequate facilities near your office for the transfer of sick or disabled persons. This becomes especially important during bad weather.
- *Poor public transportation.* Provide bus, train, and subway information, and give the phone numbers of reliable taxi companies that provide service to your office. This can be published in a handout leaflet, or in your patient newsletter.

Problem 2:
Realistic Access

Goal 1: Make sure your office is realistically accessible to all patients.

Strategies: Many patients with chronic diseases find it difficult, if not impossible, to get to your office, and follow-up care for them can become a problem. Some doctors believe that they can't provide care if the patient can't come to the office. But many services can be provided to ensure continuity of care, and to keep those patients in your practice. For example:

- Provide transportation to and from your office for invalids or housebound patients. In many communities, volunteer groups welcome the opportunity to pick up and deliver patients who can't otherwise get to medical appointments. There is usually a minimal fee, or a yearly contribution to the organization.
- Assign an office nurse to make periodic home visits to hypertensives for blood pressure checks, to diabetics for blood sugar checks, and to homebound patients for general evaluations.

Goal 2: Evaluate possible benefits from locating a satellite office closer to a target segment of current and/or potential patients.

Strategies:
- Conduct surveys to find the geographic locations and common demographic characteristics of patients who are now inconvenienced by your office location.
- Evaluate the cost-effectiveness of a satellite office in that area, considering anticipated patient load, expenses, and your personal cost and inconvenience.

Many physicians, especially those who have been in practice for several years, find that their patients have migrated from their practice area. Although many of the faithful will travel a good distance to see you, keep one startling statistic in mind: More than half of all patients change doctors every six years. This erosion of patient loyalty is expected to become even more extensive. So when a large percentage of your current practice has moved, your decision may be to relocate the entire office, or to open a satellite. The expense of opening and operating a satellite office is considerable, but in the long run it may be more cost-effective than moving.

Problem 3:
Referral Access

Goal: Evaluate the possibility of relocating your services to make them more convenient to physicians who refer patients to you, and to those patients.

Strategies:
- Project the cost and potential practice growth in relocating your office, or setting up a satellite referral office, closer to your referral base.
- Try sharing space on a part-time basis, close to the geographic center of your referral system.

In many areas, referral physicians have migrated with the population, leaving many specialists behind—surgeons, ophthalmologists, obstetricians, among others. If the majority of your specialty practice is office-based, or when your referrals are more apt to go to a more convenient physician, your decision to move becomes crucial. It must be based on sound studies that indicate whether you can survive in your current location by relying on new referring physicians.

Problem 4:
Stagnation
Your practice is in a stagnant area. No growth is projected, and your patient base is drying up.

Goal: Explore growing areas for possible extension or relocation of practice.

Strategies:
- Review available demographic data to gauge current and anticipated growth areas in the community.
- Evaluate the benefits and costs of relocating or expanding into potential growth areas.

No physician wants to go through the hassle of moving, especially if he or she has a large, established practice. Growth, however, depends on a steady influx of new patients, and if those patients can't get to your office easily, you have a serious marketing problem. We'll discuss techniques to alleviate that problem in the next chapter. But what if the competition has already moved into the growth areas? Your chances of attracting those patients are slim.

If your location has served you well for many years, but no longer will support growth, you could maintain your small yet dependable patient base right where you are—and open a satellite office in the center of the growth area.

AVAILABILITY
STRATEGIES
Even if you've corrected any accessibility problems, you may still need to face one or more of these four problems with your availability.

Problem 1:
Inconvenient Hours
Your patients feel your office hours make it inconvenient or even impossible for them to get to you when they need to and can.

Goal: Evaluate and restructure your hours for the convenience of your current and potential patients.

Strategies:
■ Keep the office open later to attract working people.
■ Open several nights a week.
■ Open earlier so parents can bring sick children in before work.
■ Maintain part-time hours on weekends to keep patients who might otherwise go to freestanding clinics.
■ Stagger your office coverage so that one physician works earlier and goes home earlier. One could work, say, from 7 a.m. to 3 p.m., another from 11 a.m. to 7 p.m.

The question of convenient office hours is complex. How much should a practice cater to the convenience of the patient? Do physicians have to work longer, more varied hours in order to survive?

The answers depend on individual marketing problems. An established but growing practice may be able to continue its current policy and survive. Practices that are struggling to survive under their current policies may have to restructure their hours. Whether the strains of competition will eventually force everyone into longer workweeks, we can't predict. But it will be more and more a luxury for doctors to stick, hard and fast, only to daytime office hours.

Problem 2:
Patients Wait Too Long
Patients have to wait too long for appointments, and then too long in your reception area.

Goal: Give patients appointments within a reasonable time, and cut waiting time in reception area.

Strategies:
- Improve scheduling to ensure time is available each day for patients requiring immediate attention.
- Ensure that patients get prompt appointments, or explanations for long delays.
- Re-evaluate current system to see why patients are waiting so long in reception area.
- Construct a patient flowchart pinpointing the times patients get to the office, are checked in at the front desk, are escorted to an examining room, and are finally seen by you. This will help you identify the bottlenecks.
- Improve patients' perception of waiting time by providing health-care brochures, interesting magazines, music, and/or audiovisual programs in the reception area. This satisfies patient desires for more health information, and also helps them pass the time.

Problem 3:
No Phone Contact
Patients are dissatisfied because they can't reach you by phone during the day.

Goal: Improve your phone availability without totally disrupting your day.

Strategies:
- Ask the phone company to conduct a free utilization survey to pinpoint peak times of phone use by your office.
- Use this data to help evaluate staff problems in dealing with telephone calls.
- Have impartial parties call your office asking for appointments. Set a variety of scenarios, such as a new family in town and a critically sick patient. Gauge staff reactions.
- Establish a protocol for phone calls, specifying which are to be answered immediately and which can be returned later in the day.
- Set aside several periods each day to return calls. Have the staff notify each patient when you can be expected to return their calls.
- Never, never fail to return a call. If an emergency occurs, have a staff member call the patient and explain why you will be delayed.
- Let a nurse screen calls and handle minor medical questions.
- Leave at least one phone line to the office open during lunch, or give the caller a prerecorded number to call in case of an emergency.
- Publish all established policies on phone calls for the benefit of both staff and patients.

The failure to handle phone calls efficiently gives the impression of a doctor too busy to care. Most patients are willing to wait if they know the call will be returned.

Problem 4:
No After-Hours Contact
Patients are dissatisfied with lack of after-hours availability.

Goal: Ensure coverage 24 hours a day, with calls handled quickly and efficiently.

Strategies:
- Conduct a survey to pinpoint specific problems patients have with your after-hours coverage.
- Evaluate your on-call system to make sure there are no time gaps when you or your partners are not available.
- Get from your answering service a list of all calls that came in on a particular night, and on at least one weekend. Have a staff person call each patient and ask if the calls were returned promptly.
- Post on-call policies in a prominent spot in your office.
- When a patient needs you after hours, make sure you see him or her.
- When you're called by a referring physician to see a patient, see that patient—day or night. Otherwise, your referring doctor will simply find someone else the next time help is needed.

Many physicians tell patients, "Go to the emergency room." That may be more convenient for the doctor, but it's seen by patients as simply uncaring. And they may quickly decide that if you won't see them at night, maybe they should find a doctor who will.

A specialist is often typed as a doctor who will see you during the day, but who is difficult to reach at night. If your referral base is not completely established, you'd better make sure you get out of bed to take care of people.

Summary
Physicians have traditionally delivered their services when and where they wanted. So the place component of your marketing mix may be hard to adjust to. But doctors who cling to the old practice of just hanging out a shingle anywhere, and expecting the patients to keep on coming, may soon find their practices failing. Patients know whether it's hard to get your services at the right time and place. So if you don't meet their accessibility needs, the comparative convenience offered by your competitors may eventually draw away many of your patients. And you'll never know how many potential patients decided not to come to you.

Reference

1. Hillestad SG, Berkowitz EN: *Health Care Marketing Plans: From Strategy to Action*. Homewood, IL: Dow Jones-Irwin, 1984.

CHAPTER 12

They won't know you're there if you don't tell them

The final P of the marketing mix, Promotion, is the element that provokes the most controversy. The widely used definitions of promotion clash with the traditional views of medicine. So before anything else, it's vitally important to understand and realistically appreciate what ethical promotion *can* and *should* be. Without it, having a quality *product* in the right *place* at the right time and at the right *price* won't help you very much.

When asked to give a quick definition of marketing, many answer, "advertising." But that's like equating antibiotics with penicillin. It's mistaking a part for the whole. Each part of the marketing mix is effective when properly entered, but in many instances other elements are equally or more effective. Promotion, as we'll discuss shortly, encompasses many communication factors. Advertising is only one of them.

Actually, *communication* is a more embracing term for what we're talking about, since it includes all methods of relaying information about your services to both current and potential patients. It's the cornerstone of any successful marketing service,

Figure 12-A
MARKETING COMMUNICATION ELEMENTS

Source:	Channel:	Receiver:
• Physician	• Practice Newsletter	• Present Patients
• Group Practice	• Paid Advertising	• Potential Patients
• Specialty Association	• Newspaper Column	• Referral Physicians
	• Personal Conversations	• Employers
		• Health Plans

but it's even more important in the intensely personal service of health care.

CHANNELS OF PROMOTION The function of promotion is to let people know that you have a quality product, competitively priced, and accessible to them. In short, you must get the word out.

All communication—all promotion—involves three elements: a *source*, a *channel*, and a *receiver*. *(See Fig. 12-A)*

The *source* is the person or business initiating the information flow. It may be an individual (a doctor), a group (two or more doctors), or an institution (a specialty association). In marketing, the source may use many forms: a printed or electronic message, such as a logotype or sign; a spoken message; or a simple, nonverbal message, such as empathy, attentiveness, or bedside manner.

The *channel* is the medium. It may be a practice newsletter, a paid advertisement, a newspaper column, or—most importantly—conversations that you or your staff have with others. The channel may also be the source—the person used to carry the message, say, a physician communicating with a patient.

The *receiver* is the object of the message. Current and potential patients, other physicians, employers, and health plans can all be receivers of your message.

Promotion is any means used to inform, remind, or persuade customers about a product or service. It can be done directly by contact with the customer, or indirectly through intermediaries—referring physicians, for example. It can be used to induce an immediate or long-range response. When a department store holds an "After Christmas Sale," it wants people to flock in on a specific day or days.

A different promotional strategy is often used by oil companies. They speak of energy conservation, and attempt to build long-term good will to enhance both their corporate image and, by association, their products. They emphasize an issue, rather than the virtues of a specific product.

Traditionally, the issue-oriented approach has been the promotional strategy of the medical profession, as epitomized by the AMA and other professional groups and societies. What's good for medicine is what's good for doctors.

That's certainly true. But today, it's not enough. A number of competitors in the health-care field are marketing so strenuously for the immediate customer that their efforts sometimes resemble a fire sale. While many physicians wouldn't want even vaguely to imitate this extreme, there's a middle ground that allows both effective promotion and adherence to professional ethics. In this chapter we'll examine three kinds of ethical promotion: *personal selling, public relations,* and *advertising.* We'll show you how you can use these tools without fearing the wrath of the ethics committee.

Personal Selling

In marketing terms, "personal selling" is a face to face, oral presentation to prospective customers in order to persuade them to buy your product or service. Such a blunt definition will make a lot of sensitive physicians cringe.

Most doctors are turned off by the idea of selling, yet every one of us does some personal selling almost every day, whether or not we know it or want to admit it. You sell every time you talk with a patient or a referral doctor, or when you speak to a group. And what you sell helps make tangible one major intangible product—yourself.

Public Relations

P.R. involves building and maintaining sound bonds with a number of specific "publics." For doctors, those publics include patients, businesses, industry, and even government agencies.

Traditionally, most medical organizations have paid little attention to public relations. The attitude was that physicians are required to do a lot of community service, but no one is supposed to know about it. That's not to say that everything a doctor does should be featured on the 6 o'clock news. But why keep good works a secret?

If you believe in what you're doing, and you're providing quality medical care, shouldn't you be proud, and even obligated, to tell others? Good P.R. can enhance a physician's image, and that can improve the patients' perceptions of quality, which in turn translates directly into practice growth.

The trend now is for physicians to hire professional P.R. firms to "build an image."[1] But using public relations doesn't necessitate hiring anyone. Good, ethical P.R. can be as easy as sending out a brief news release when you or your practice accomplishes something for the good of the community.

A group practice on the West Coast, for example, became concerned about the incidence of high blood pressure in a poor section of town. The doctors spent several weekends taking free B.P. checks and referring those with elevated levels to the community health center. Those same physicians also donated much of their spare time as consultants to a new hypertension clinic. As an afterthought, an aggressive business manager asked the local newspaper if it would be interested in a story. The editor jumped at the idea. The ethical, tasteful article that followed not only improved medicine's image; it increased patient referrals to the practice.

Advertisements

An ad is one way an identified, paying sponsor can communicate an idea about goods and services to a mass audience. The objectives of advertising are to introduce a product or service, enter a new market, and reach potential buyers it would be too costly to reach otherwise. The objectives of your particular ad are to increase awareness of, increase interest in, generate a trial of, or hasten adoption of your particular product or service.

The advertising message is referred to as *copy*. When considering the effectiveness of your copy, take into account how the message is conveyed, how it's designed, and how it's seen by the consumer. The channels through which copy is conveyed are the media—including newspapers, magazines, telephone directories, radio, television, and billboards.

Roots of Medical Advertising

Both the moral and economic justification for advertising stems from its ability to increase competition in the selling of a particular product or service, which in turn tends to reduce the cost to the consumer.

Few physicians considered advertising until the 1977 Supreme Court case of *Bates and O'Steen v. the State Bar of Arizona,* a decision affirming the right of attorneys to advertise. This decision opened the path for any professional to advertise without fear of legal ostracism by colleagues. This landmark case also added fuel to Federal Trade Commission allegations of restraint of trade by health-care organizations, specifically the American Medical Association and the American Dental Association.

For many years, based on its law-enforcement duties in the realm of antitrust and consumer protection, the FTC felt it had jurisdiction over the activities of organizations such as the AMA. In 1979, after many years of debate, the FTC found the AMA and other medical organizations engaging in illegal conspiracies to restrict competition. The commission cited the AMA Code of Ethics that restricted its members from advertising. It ruled that these restrictions posed "unethical" restraints on doctors' truthful advertising to inform consumers.

The FTC cited the example of a county medical society that used restrictions to hinder a church-sponsored program providing low-cost tests to detect heart disease. In another case, the FTC cited advertising restrictions used to help drive a physician house-call group out of business.

Revised Medical Ethics. The 1979 FTC order was appealed, but was upheld by the Second Circuit Court of Appeals in 1980, and again by the Supreme Court in 1982. That final decision led to revision of the AMA's "Principles of Medical Ethics." The opinion of the AMA Judicial Council now states, "There are no restrictions on advertising by physicians except those that can be specifically justified to protect the public from deceptive practices."[2] The council also attempted to further define the form and content of ethical advertising.

The new guidelines allow a physician to advertise through any channel: newspapers, magazines, telephone directories, radio, television, handbills, billboards, even skywriting. The only restrictions are that the copy not be misleading, false, or deceptive. The communication may include (a) the educational background of the physician, (b) the basis on which fees are determined, (c) available credit or other methods of payment, and (d) other information about the physician that a reasonable person might regard as relevant in choosing the doctor's services. *(See Fig. 12-B)*

What was the FTC trying to accomplish? According to Carol T. Crawford, director of the FTC's Bureau of Consumer Protection, "Physician advertising can be an important spur to competition, a low-cost way to inform the public, and an incentive for professionals to design different ways to deliver health care."[3]

FTC Chairman James C. Miller III said, "A rigorous and competitive marketplace will help consumers." The FTC was apparently following the traditional business assumption that advertising will ultimately promote competition and lower costs.

Despite all of those actions, the incidence of advertising by fee-for-service physicians is still low. Various observers, however, expect it to increase dramatically as the competitive medical marketplace continues to heat up.

Figure 12-B
ADVERTISING AND PUBLICITY

5.01 There are no restrictions on advertising by physicians except those that can be specifically justified to protect the public from deceptive practices. A physician may publicize himself as a physician through any commercial publicity or other form of public communication (including any newspaper, magazine, telephone directory, radio, television or other advertising) provided that the communication shall not be misleading because of the omission of necessary material information, shall not contain any false or misleading statement, or shall not otherwise operate to deceive.

The form of communication should be designed to communicate the information contained therein to the public in a direct, dignified, and readily comprehensible manner. Aggressive, high pressure advertising and publicity may create unjustified medical expectations. Any advertisement or publicity, regardless of format or content should be true and not misleading.

The communication may include: (a) the educational background of the physician; (b) the basis on which fees are determined (including charges for specific services); (c) available credit or other methods of payment; and (d) other information about the physician which a reasonable person might regard as relevant in determining whether to seek the physician's services.

Testimonials of patients, however, as to the physician's skill or the quality of his professional services should not be publicized. Statements relating to the quality of medical services are extremely difficult, if not impossible, to verify or measure by objective standards. Claims regarding experience, competence, and the quality of the physician's services may be made if they can be factually supported and if they do not imply that he has an exclusive and unique skill or remedy. A statement that a physician has cured or successfully treated a large number of cases involving a particular serious ailment may imply a certainty of result and create unjustified and misleading expectations in prospective patients.

Consistent with Federal regulatory standards which apply to commercial advertising, a physician who is considering the placement of an advertisement or publicity release, whether in print, radio, or television, should determine in advance that his communication or message is explicitly and implicitly truthful and not misleading. These standards require the advertiser to have a reasonable basis for claims before they are used in advertising. The reasonable basis must be established by those facts known to the advertiser, and those which a reasonable, prudent advertiser should have discovered.

As used herein, reference to a "physician" applies also to information relating to the physician's group, partners or associates. Any communication or message within the scope of this opinion should include the name of at least one physician responsible for its content.

Source: "Current Opinions of the Judicial Council of the American Medical Association" (1982)

Figure 12-C
COMMUNICATION TRIANGLE

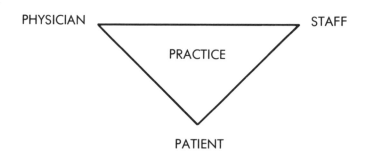

RINGING THE
COMMUNICATION TRIANGLE
In the medical-exchange process, communication primarily occurs among physician, patient, and staff. Therefore, improving your communication skills, and those of your staff, should be priority goals.

There are three channels to be developed before effective communication can take place. All are equal in importance, and each must complement the others. We call it the "Communication Triangle"—doctor-patient, doctor-staff, and staff-patient. *(See Fig. 12-C)*

Physician-Patient
Communication
We've said it before, but it can't be emphasized enough: Patients want and need better communication with their doctors. Even when communication does occur, it's too often in the language of "medicalese." Patients also often feel physicians are too busy to listen to their concerns and fears. If physicians expect patients to remain with them, they must deal with any patients' perceptions of them as "poor communicators."

Communicators' Keys. Have you ever dealt with people you felt were excellent communicators? What skills did they have? You probably recall that they:
- Made you feel they were focusing on your every word.
- Spoke clearly, briefly, and directly.
- Encouraged you to express your opinions.
- Left you feeling they were unhurried, no matter how busy they really were.

The next time you talk with a patient, review those skills in your mind to see if you truly have them. If you don't, begin to develop techniques to tap or improve them.

Ten Commandments of Communication.

I. Don't hurry; make the patient feel he or she is the only one you have to think about at that moment.

II. Open each encounter with: "It's good to see you again," not, "Why are you here today?" Your session with the patient should include a lot of eye contact and good, active listening.

III. Hold the opening encounter, no matter how brief, when the patient is dressed. That provides the opportunity to meet you initially on more comfortable terms. Walking in on a draped patient may make for quicker visits, but people then think of you as a doctor who's too busy to talk with them.

IV. Communicate with the patient on physically equal terms. Many physicians stand while talking with seated patients. This is seen as an authoritarian pose. It's the way policemen interrogate suspects, towering over them, intimidating them physically and psychologically. An aware physician doesn't do this. Instead, place two small chairs in each examining room so you can sit close and be on the same level as the patient.

V. Ask, "Is there anything else you're concerned about?" That gives the patient an opportunity to express any inner anxieties.

VI. Don't interrupt an encounter with a phone call, unless absolutely necessary. "If he's that busy," thinks the patient, "maybe I should go elsewhere."

VII. End each meeting with, "It was good to see you. Thank you for coming." If the patient is sick, add, "I'm concerned about you, so call tomorrow and let me know how you're doing."

VIII. End each meeting by being sure the patient understands what's been done, why it was done, what's been found, and what the treatment will be. Many times, physicians assume that patients understand, rather than making sure they do.

IX. Provide oral and written instructions, and when possible, back those up with printed educational material, such as a brochure on high blood pressure.

X. Listen to your patients. Pay particular attention to nonverbal clues, such as anger because of underlying fear.

Patient-Staff Communication
No matter how effective you are in dealing with patients, all your good efforts can be ruined by a quick or curt remark delivered by a thoughtless staff member. Patients hold

the physician directly responsible for the actions of the staff. They're as likely to change doctors because of bad staff attitudes as because of dissatisfaction with you. There are four critical areas of staff interaction with patients: *telephone, scheduling, nursing,* and *collections.*

Phoning. Physicians are concerned that their nursing staff be of the highest quality, and they want people with a lot of experience to handle the business side of the practice. But many physicians think of other staff jobs as rather lowly and capable of being done by almost anyone. Yet, answering a physician's phone is a difficult job requiring a great deal of skill and maturity.

We once heard a receptionist answer the phone by saying, "No, Ms. Jones, you can't talk with the doctor, he's much too busy for you." Pause. "Yes, I'll try and get him to call you back, but you know today is his day off and sometimes I can't get him to return calls."

Too often, in trying to protect their employer, receptionists end up hurting both the doctor and the practice. Here are six approaches to making your telephone a positive marketing tool:

1. In your next staff meeting, emphasize that phone calls are not just a necessary evil in your employees' daily routines, but a major reason for their employment.
2. Remind staff that most patients are sick and frightened when they call, and therefore anxious and ultrasensitive.
3. Reassure patients that their calls will be answered, and give them some idea of when. Work out some preset times each day when you answer calls, and make sure patients know those times. That avoids the inconsiderate practice of making them wait all day for you to call.
4. Tell patients that you welcome their calls and will be accessible to them.
5. If a patient is told that the call will be returned, return it, or else have staff notify the caller why there will be a delay. One physician makes sure when he's on duty in the OB suite during the day, that all calls are returned by the receptionist, giving each patient a new time when he'll be able to call back.
6. Empathizing with patients is part of the job of every staff member, especially the receptionist. Responding to an anxious patient with, "You sound as if you really feel badly, so let me get this message to the doctor quickly," may not get the call answered any faster, but it gives the impression that your people care.

Scheduling. An efficient appointments secretary is a precious commodity. The ability to give a patient the feeling of being cared for in every way is a great gift. But many patients complain that they can't get an appointment when they want one. Offering to book them in earlier if there's a cancellation is an effective way to let patients know you're doing everything you can to work around their schedules.

Telling a patient with a high fever and a cough on Monday that the doctor can't see him or her until next Friday is a major blunder. It's far better to say, "I'm concerned that you're really sick; let me check with the doctor and see when we can work you in."

Nursing. Patients become irritated when they're given the old response by the nurse: "Wait till you see the doctor; he'll tell you what you need to know." Patients deserve to know what is done by the nursing staff. It's reasonable to expect the nursing staff to show concern and to go out of their way to explain what's going on. Including the nurse as an integral part of the communication team will ease the time pressures on you.

Collecting. From the moment the patient enters the office, the whole practice should be centered on him or her. Once the visit is over, however, the emphasis is on paying for the services. The way staff relates to a patient when attempting to collect for the visit may have a lot to do with how that patient views the total experience. Try to understand and always sympathize with the patient, but be firm in your business policies.

Physician-Staff Communication

In several practice surveys, we found major problems that were rooted in poor communication between physicians and staffs. Successful marketing requires staff members not only to understand what's going on, but to feel a part of the whole process. Physicians must communicate their goals for the practice, and how they feel those goals should be met. In turn, they should be willing to listen to staff suggestions and criticisms. Many times, the people who deal day by day with a particular problem have a better appreciation of how it can be solved.

We've always felt that physicians need to have a better reading of what their staff does. So look at their jobs from their points of view, not yours. Listen to their frustrations. Hold regular meetings with staff and give them the opportunity to criticize without fear of losing their jobs.

The concept of quality circles, mentioned earlier as a Japanese innovation, could certainly be applied to health care. As practiced by industry, these circles are small groups of employees who meet regularly to discuss how they can make their firm more quality oriented.

In effect, an enlightened physician can turn his staff meetings into quality circles.

PRINT TOOLS OF YOUR TRADE

In addition to effective interpersonal skills, good communication can be achieved through printed material. It can give current and potential patients permanent resource material to refer to when questions arise about your practice. It's also an excellent means for providing general health information.

Your Calling Card: A Practice Brochure

One of the best ways to relay information to the patient is through a practice brochure. To be effective, your brochure should:

■ Clearly reveal the principles of your practice.

■ Create an image of warmth and caring.

■ Tell current and potential patients what your specialty and services are all about.

■ Detail your practice, policies, and procedures.

■ Reflect concern both for the people already in your practice, and for those considering entry.

To accomplish those goals, you need to present the following nine items of information, clearly and concisely:

1. A message that reflects your concern for your patients.
2. A thank you to them for their trust in you.
3. A statement of your philosophy of medical practice, including your views on health maintenance and regular physicals.
4. Your office hours, address, and phone number, answering service and emergency numbers. Some brochures include a map with directions to the office.
5. How to make an appointment, how long it might take, how quickly they can expect to be seen if they're suddenly sick, what to do and where to go in an emergency.
6. How and when their calls will be answered.
7. How fees are set, and how you handle health insurance and collections.
8. A brief list of the qualifications of the doctors.
9. Details of the specialty and services offered.

A practice brochure may be quite elaborate with bound copy on glossy paper, or it may be relatively simple with $8\frac{1}{2}$-by-11-inch paper folded in thirds. The format you choose will depend on the money and time you want to spend. But your brochure must be of good quality because it is a projection of you and your practice.

Distribute it at least expense by third-class bulk mailing. Be sure to have copies of your brochure in the office for new patients and their friends and family members not on your mailing list.

Practice brochures are highly effective marketing tools that can often help clarify points of misunderstanding. If left unaddressed, those small misunderstandings can easily grow and lead to great patient dissatisfaction.

Practice Newsletter

During the past decade, the American public has expressed an increasing interest in health care. Marketing surveys point to education as a primary desire of most patients, yet they're getting a major portion of such information from the popular print and electronic media. Those same surveys indicate that patients want—and in many cases, prefer—this information to come from their physicians. In fact, not providing this information is seen as a major weakness of doctors.

Since physicians must accept the responsibility for educating their patients in a meaningful manner, the practice newsletter is an effective way to get the information across to them. It's also an excellent marketing tool.

Beginning. You may feel that a practice newsletter is too great an undertaking. But it needn't take much time, and even in a small practice, much of the responsibility can be shared with the staff.

The most important requirement is that the information be relevant to your patients and your practice. In the beginning, this may include asking a selected group of patients what kinds of information they would like to read. This also involves making sure it's timely. An article on preventing cramps when swimming will not be well received in the fall, nor will the details on flu vaccine have a big audience in midsummer. (We'll cover more on timeliness under *Seasonal health problems* below.)

The Content Quartet. Before beginning to prepare copy, plan exactly what you want to include. A good approach is for your first newsletter to have four separate sections that can become permanent parts of future editions. They may be called by any titles you choose, but should include the following:

1. *Practice information.* Give your office policies and procedures. You might cover office hours, business policies, and new services. You might also answer common questions that you and your staff are asked about the practice and its services.

2. *Preventive health care.* This tells patients how to stay healthy. Suggestions on proper diet, exercise, and cancer prevention are exceptionally well received. By informing patients about health-related issues, and by increasing their awareness of potential health problems, you're encouraging them to seek medical attention and to get it from you. From a marketing point of view, this section can serve as a means of advising patients of the importance of staying healthy, and using your practice as a tool to achieve that goal.

3. *Self-help health tips.* Patients not only want general health information. They want to know how to take care of themselves so that they don't get sick, and how to provide some of their own care when they do. For a primary-care physician, the information might include how to take care of fever, diarrhea, a nonproductive cough, and common cuts. The more you help your patients learn about self care, the more healthy and appreciative they'll be—and the more they'll use your services when they're really needed. It will also result in fewer unnecessary office visits and phone calls. All in all, providing self-help aid is an excellent example of sound ethics wedded to sound marketing.

4. *Seasonal health problems.* This section should discuss problems relevant to the time of year. The fall issue might include an article on the flu and the need for certain people to have the vaccine. The spring issue could deal with allergies, the summer issue with sunburn and poison ivy. This section can also show some of the ways your practice can help with those specific problems, and serve as a "hook" to get patients into the office for flu shots and other treatment.

Though the above information pertains basically to primary-care physicians, referral physicians can also use newsletters to good advantage. An orthopedist could send a biannual or quarterly newsletter to current and potential referring physicians on topics such as how to diagnose and treat common knee injuries. An ophthalmologist could do the same on common eye injuries, or proper diagnosis of glaucoma.

The purpose of sending your practice newsletter to referring physicians is threefold:

■ Identifies you as a concerned specialist willing to help educate other physicians in your area of expertise.

■ Helps other doctors understand your specialty and how it meshes with that of the primary physician.

■ Shows that you are accessible and welcome more referrals when other doctors need the services of your specialty.

Figure 12-D

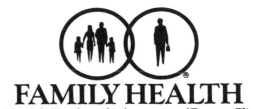

FAMILY HEALTH
A Quarterly Newsletter for the patients of **Decatur Clinic.**

Healthy Lifestyles
The True Flu

Influenza, or the flu, is a specific viral illness whose symptoms include general body aches, headaches, sore throat, dry cough, and a runny nose. Unlike a cold, the flu can also cause nausea, weakness and high fever.

Type A virus is the most common form of influenza, causing epidemics across the nation about every three years. Our bodies can build up immunity against future attacks, but the virus itself keeps changing. Outbreaks of Type B influenza virus are not as widespread and occur about every ten years.

In susceptible individuals, immunization is the surest way to prevent the flu. This means getting one shot sometime in October or November just before the flu season begins. People in good health don't need flu shots, but it is extremely important for those who are **over 65** or who have **heart disease** or **respiratory problems.** Other high risk candidates for whom immunization is recom-

mended are **diabetics,** people who are **anemic,** those with **kidney disease,** and **post-operative patients.** This immunization only works against Type A and Type B influenza. The flu shot will not protect you from any other type of virus. Any high risk candidate should contact their doctor if they contract the flu. If you are not at risk, you should contact the doctor if you are not getting better in 2-3 days or if you are running a fever for more than 48-72 hours.

Antibiotics are useless against the flu. The only way to be more comfortable is to fight the symptoms with aspirin or acetaminophen for the aches and fever. Cough syrups and decongestants may also be helpful. Remember to rest and drink plenty of fluids.

Your Family Doctor

The family doctor has met the health needs of families for generations. Today, your family physician is a specialist in the field of medicine or family practice. This is the specialty in modern medicine that emphasizes comprehensive medical care with special attention to the family unit.

The family physician is educated and trained in a unique way. The attitudes and skills which are developed qualify the family practice physician to provide continuing health maintenance and medical care to the entire family from infancy to maturity.

The education of the family physician follows the general practice tradition, but has some major differences. Upon completion of medical school and before entering practice, the physician must complete a three-year residency training program. In addition to broad hospital-based inpatient training, family physicians receive extensive training in outpatient medicine for all ages. Their training combines the content of other clinical disciplines such as internal medicine, pediatrics, obstetrics and gynecology, surgery, behavioral sciences and preventive medicine. These are integrated into a single specialty with a focus on patient care in the context of the family community. With this background the family doctor can serve as the patient or family advocate and advisor in all health-related matters and in the appropriate use of consultants, other medical specialists and community resources.

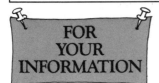

FOR YOUR INFORMATION

The physicians of Decatur Clinic present the first edition of Family Health, a quarterly newsletter for their patients. In an effort to keep our patients aware of current health topics and informed of changes, information is provided to assist the Clinic's new patients and those who have been seeing our doctors on a regular basis throughout the years.

It is our hope that this newsletter and forthcoming issues will answer some of your questions and provide you with useful information. As always, the doctors and staff of Decatur Clinic are available to meet the needs of you and your family.

Change of Address: Decatur Clinic has another change of address, BUT NOT LOCATION. The City of Decatur has changed the name of Columbia Drive to Commerce Drive. Some of you will remember our former office on Ponce de Leon, and have been to the Columbia Drive location. To avoid any confusion when asking for directions, we have not relocated, but have had our street address changed. This new address, 755 Commerce Drive, will be reflected on your new statements and future correspondence.
Insurance: As in the past, Decatur Clinic does not accept any assignment of benefits from insurance companies on behalf of our patients. Your insurance carrier has a contract with you, and that business contract should not enter the Physician/patient relationship. We do, however, communicate with your carriers to provide them with information that will expedite payment of your claims. In the near future, our secretaries will be asking for some information from you about your insurance to help us more adequately answer any questions the carriers may ask us. This does not affect the current policy regarding the

responsibility of the patient to pursue their own insurance carriers.

A key word in most contracts is "deductible." The deductible is that portion of your claims which you pay before your insurance begins to pay. Even though your current visit may not exceed your contract deductible, you should file a claim so the carrier can begin accumulating these charges toward meeting your deductible. Of course, once your deductible has been met, your insurance will pay those claims appropriately covered under your particular contract.

Telephone Tips: In the past, we have encountered several problems regarding which telephone number to use and when. Each of the doctors has several incoming lines indicated on your appointment card. The business office can be reached by calling **377-6424.** By utilizing the direct doctor line, your call does not have to be forwarded through the business office and can be handled faster. If you need to contact a doctor after office hours for an emergency, our doctor on call can be reached at **898-0411.**

Developing the Text. The next step is getting all that information down on paper. Many doctors throw up their hands at this point, because they feel they don't have writing talent. It's surprising that doctors spend a great part of their day relating health information to patients, yet feel they can't convey the same information in written form. Nonsense. With very little effort, physicians can learn to put it on paper. Here are a few suggestions:

■ Talk out what you want into your dictating machine.

■ Say it as if you were speaking to an eighth-grade student, using words that the majority of your patients understand.

■ Get a secretary to type it out.

■ Ask a member of your staff with talent and interest in writing, and a few candid, nonmedical friends to critique the content and make sure it's understandable and interesting.

Packaging. After you've gathered your articles, decide how you want the newsletter to look. Do you want it to be one or two columns wide? Will you use the logo from your stationery, or design one specially for the newsletter? What kind of typeface do you want? You may decide to do it "typewriter" style, a common newsletter format. Or you can let a printer do the designing and typesetting. Figure 12-D is a sample of a successful practice newsletter. Printing and mailing costs and procedures are laid out in Appendix E.

Patient Education

Physicians who refuse to respond to the interest in "do-it-yourself" health care will have difficulty retaining and acquiring patients. There are many ways to respond. The methods will depend somewhat on your type of practice. An obstetrician will impart different information than an ophthalmologist. Here are some methods oriented toward specific informational needs.

Test Information. Patients need to know more about tests performed on them. Laboratory, X-ray, and other diagnostic tests you order should be explained in detail. This puts patients at ease, and helps them form a better impression of you.

Patient handouts are easy to prepare. The best way is to start with some of your most commonly performed tests and develop a "fact sheet." This would include what the test attempts to establish, why it was ordered, what the patient can expect from the test, how much it costs, and what you will do with the results. The following is the kind of information a test "fact sheet" should contain:

"What is an IVP? The abbreviation IVP stands for intravenous pyelography, an examination in which X-rays are taken of the kidneys

and other organs of the urinary tract. *Intravenous*, meaning 'within a vein,' refers to the injection of the contrast medium, which darkens the urine and allows the hollow internal structures of the urinary tract to be visualized. *Pyelo-* refers to the 'renal pelvis,' a part of the kidney. The suffix *-graphy*, meaning 'writing' or 'picture,' refers to the X-rays taken during IVP.''

Drug Information. Medication is perhaps the subject patients are most interested in. They want to know why a medicine is ordered, what it will do, what the side effects are, if there are any interactions with other medicines they're taking, and if a generic equivalent is available.

The most obvious way to provide information about medications is for you, or a member of your staff, to sit down with patients and explain each drug prescribed. This solution is ideal, but many doctors aren't prepared to spend the time. Rather than ignore the need, consider using more drug-information handouts. Currently, the AMA, through its Patient Medication Instruction program, and the American Academy of Family Physicians, through its Drug Use Education Tips program, have developed excellent fact sheets on a wide variety of commonly used drugs. After prescribing a particular medication, follow up with a brief discussion on why the drug was ordered, and give the patient a drug fact sheet to take home.

Disease Information. Why do physicians assume patients have a doctoral degree in disease? Many patients complain that their doctors will tell them what's wrong, but that's all. Patients want more information about what the disease or problem is all about, what they can expect in terms of recovery, what disabilities they might develop, and what the chances are of having the problem again.

Physicians have many brochures at their fingertips that explain about particular diseases or health problems in language that patients can understand. Doctors should develop libraries of disease-oriented brochures to cover their specialties.

Audio-Visuals. Today's consumers are audio-visually oriented. Take advantage of that and develop A/V facilities. Many physicians are now setting aside a room with A/V equipment where a patient can learn about a disease or a surgical procedure that's been recommended. During the viewing, you can see other patients and then return to answer questions the video may have sparked.

Computers. Consumers are also turning to the computer for help in performing many of their daily tasks. Computer programs can teach patients self-help, and provide information on preventive medicine and drugs. There are programs that tell consumers what might be wrong with them after descriptions of symptoms have been fed into the computer. Imagine patients calling your office, not with symptoms, but with a diagnosis, and even with a computer recommendation for treatment.

You can use patient-oriented software in your office computer. You can also provide patients with personalized hard-copy information through the computer's word processing feature. You might even lend patients software to take home and use with their own computers.

Summary

This chapter has built the foundation for a more specific discussion of how you can pragmatically, yet ethically, promote your practice. The next chapter examines the ethics and tactics of promotion strategies.

References

1. Hull JB: The doc's on TV, maybe it's because he takes the PR Rx. *Wall Street Journal*, August 23, 1983.
2. *Current Opinions of the Judicial Council of the American Medical Association.* Chicago: AMA, 1982.
3. *Medical World News*, May 28, 1984, 27.

CHAPTER 13

Promoting your practice with dignity

Some of your colleagues, perhaps even the vast majority, may tell you that marketing is unethical. Not so. But we have no intention of launching into a lengthy discourse on the subject of medical ethics. We do ask your indulgence, however, in allowing us to make just one point:

If you feel you represent the finest health-care system in the world, and if you feel that your own practice offers better total quality health care than your competitors—regardless of who they may be—and if your ultimate goal is to provide the highest quality care, then it may be unethical for you *not* to promote your practice. Why?

Because not promoting what you have to offer could deprive some potential patients of the kind of quality health care they might not get elsewhere.

During one of our recent marketing consultations, a doctor told us, "I'm a good plastic surgeon. Perhaps the best in the whole area. But I'm new. So just what does a guy have to do to get his name known?"

It's even more ominous when an excellent physician runs head on into a big corporation that can spend millions of dollars to out-position him or her in the marketplace. One doctor who was listening to our presentation on the use of ethical promotional tools finally threw up his hands. He'd had enough. "Let's be realistic," he said. "How can I compete against these huge HMOs and health corporations? They can spend millions, while I'm just making ends meet. I can't scrape up even a thousand dollars to compete. So I'm wasting my time here!"

Well, it's that doctor who most desperately needs effective and relatively inexpensive marketing tools. He can't, and shouldn't, spend thousands to compete with big business. He doesn't have to. All he need do is to understand that he has an arsenal of ethical weapons at his disposal in his fight to survive.

The battle shouldn't be fought on the turf of corporate advertising, because no physician or small group has that kind of money. The best strategy is to find a different battleground—one on which the average doctor is more comfortable. Fight them on your turf.

Our point is analagous to the situation confronting many small to medium-size firms in the business world. We can all cite many examples of small companies that are doing exceedingly well in situations where they directly or indirectly compete with large corporations.

Stay away from the "Big Buck vs. Big Buck" arena. Big corporations can afford it; you can't. Concentrate your efforts more on a community-oriented level. And remember that you may have a larger marketing staff—your patients. Use them.

WAYS AND MEANS TO
PROMOTE YOURSELF

You may not be aware of it, but every time you attend a community function, give a speech, or talk to referring physicians at the hospital, you're promoting your product to potential consumers. Promotion is simply making sure people are aware of the quality of your product, which happens to be *you*. You have your distinctive personality, your strengths and weaknesses. Find the strengths and personality traits that will help you market yourself, and then use them. If you don't know what you've got to sell, ask your family and friends for opinions. Perhaps you're a gifted speaker, or a good writer, or a natural community leader, fond of participating in service projects. Any of those talents would provide an excellent method of getting known in your community.

You may direct your efforts toward the community at large, the medical community, both the print and electronic media, your current patients, or other targets identified by your surveys.

In the Community

Here are some approaches to consider for developing a promotional marketing campaign. Remember, the purpose is to retain the patients you have, while attracting more.

Goal: Increase your involvement in the community.

Strategies:
- Join civic organizations that can give you and your practice increased exposure.
- Volunteer for public service committees, such as the United Way, Heart Fund, or School Board.
- Participate in public forums, community planning sessions, and local government meetings.
- Get to know influential community leaders, and offer your services when they can be of use.

Physicians seem to have lost their traditional role as community leaders. It can't be proven, but it makes you wonder how much this declining leadership has contributed to the declining popularity of doctors.

So get involved. We can't emphasize that too strongly. People will view your commitment as a sign of caring. What other quality is more important for a physician to project? When potential patients feel you're willing to give valuable time to the future of the place you live, they're apt to remember your name when they're looking for a doctor.

Goal: Increase the community's awareness of you and your practice.

Strategies:
- Offer free sports physicals at schools; they take time, but the feedback can be very beneficial.
- Offer to serve as the physician for school or other amateur sports teams.
- Offer to speak to civic and business groups, social and religious organizations, PTAs, and high schools.
- Participate in and contribute to fund drives of local youth organizations; your time and leadership are more important than the dollars you contribute.
- Offer medical supplies, such as bandages and antiseptics, to youth organizations, hiking or other sport associations, volunteer fire companies or first-aid groups.
- Offer care for needy families identified by a religious or other charitable organization. They might be refugees, people facing a financial crisis, or the chronically poor.

- Hold free forums on topics such as heart-disease prevention, stop-smoking campaigns, family health care, and accident prevention. This is best done in conjunction with an open house, perhaps at a school, church, or synagogue that would donate the time and space.
- Speak to people everywhere you can. Be cordial and don't be afraid to introduce yourself.

Physicians often hesitate to become known in their communities because they don't want to be seen as pushy or self-seeking. But each of the above strategies provides a worthwhile service; there's nothing wrong in being connected with them. View the use of marketing in the current competitive environment and as an opportunity to reawaken yourself to your duty—to become involved as a community leader, as well as a healer.

In the Medical Community

Real estate experts point out three things to consider when buying property: location, location, and location. The same emphasis can be given to the reasons for getting to know your fellow physicians, and for contributing to the work of medical societies and organizations: referrals, referrals, and referrals.

Goal: Increase your involvement within the medical community.

Strategies:
- Join your local medical society, go to meetings, and work on some committees.
- Become active in your hospital's work, and serve on its committees that interest you and need help.
- Attend social functions, mingle, and make yourself known to other physicians, especially those who may affect your practice.
- If you have a special area of medical or nonmedical expertise, offer to share it with other physicians in departmental meetings or in other forums.

Many of today's doctors complacently avoid involvement in the social and organizational areas of their profession. Yet the better you're known among your peers, the more times your name will come up when someone is thinking of where to send a patient.

In Print

If you have an interest in writing, many avenues are open to you. We've already discussed the impact of writing a practice newsletter. Now let's look at writing for the other print media, primarily newspapers and magazines.

Almost every community has at least a weekly paper, and almost every one of them is eager to publish a physician's view on health issues, often in a regular column. This provides medical information for the public, and a forum for explaining your philosophy of health care. Here are several approaches:

- A weekly column on health-related topics.
- A daily or weekly column of health tips.
- Letters to the editor.
- An article in a local, school, or church newspaper.

Many physicians who aren't good public speakers are very good writers. If you're not sure whether you can write well, try it. You might be pleasantly surprised.

When we brought this up at a seminar, one of the doctors protested. "No way," he said. "I can't write. I can talk to patients, but I can't write an understandable article."

That wasn't true, and eventually we proved it to him. But if you feel that way, chances are you're also wrong. To prove our thesis, try this: Explain hypertension, or any other medical problem, to a patient. When you do, have your tape recorder turned on. Limit your explanation to 10 minutes. Have the tape transcribed. Nine chances out of 10, with a little editing, you'll have a finished article. See if you have some writing or editing talent on your staff, or if your spouse might want to help.

If you're still doubtful, just keep in mind that people who edit newspapers and magazines are in the business of turning sows' ears into silk purses. All they ask is that you give them good, understandable ideas, placed in something resembling logical order. You give them that, and they'll be happy to polish your stuff to near perfection.

On Radio and TV

Today's fast-paced society receives more than half its information from radio and television. Using electronic media can provide a public service and excellent exposure for you at the same time. (We're dealing here only with using the media as a public service marketing tool. We'll discuss advertising later.)

You don't have to be a "media doc" to serve your community on the airwaves. Like newspapers and magazines, radio and television stations are looking for physicians to help gather and deliver health-related stories. They're also interested in general health topics that will appeal to a wide audience.

You can work with your local media and improve your reputation as a medical authority at the same time. Your role as a consultant or expert guest will be seen in a positive light, and it can't help but improve the image of your practice. Here are some services you can offer to radio and TV:

- Help stations verify health-related stories. Reporters are always looking for cooperative, knowledgeable people to help them in areas where they're not expert. Physicians who offer timely commentary will discover news people coming back again and again for verification and commentary on health stories.
- Develop public service announcements (PSAs).
- Prerecord 30-second and 60-second health tips.

Appendix F offers tips on how to get started with your media involvement, and how to prepare and handle yourself on the air.

Keeping Your Patients _____ Don't concentrate so hard on generating new patients, that you forget about those you now have. If they're neglected, they'll find cause to leave. Preservation is not the only reason for paying careful attention to your patients. A better reason is this: Satisfied patients are great missionaries for your practice, telling others about the fine care they receive from you. To make and keep your patients happy, set and meet these twin objectives:

Goal 1: Develop ways to improve patient satisfaction.

Strategies:
- Send birthday greetings to all patients, with something special for the pediatric crowd.
- Send some form of "thank you" to everyone who refers another patient to you. Put this information in the patient's file so you can also thank him or her personally on the next office visit.
- Send reminders to patients who are due for annual checkups, Pap smears, or blood-pressure checks. Follow each reminder with a personal call from you or a member of your staff. Dentists have been doing this for years, and their patients like it.
- Periodically reward patients who lose weight, stop smoking, or keep their appointments for blood-pressure checks. Give them special praise or recognition, reduce your regular charge, or make no charge at all for that visit. The money you lose will be more than made up for by the good word of mouth and the referrals that result.
- Offer patients a pleasant reception area with beverages, current periodicals, and music or TV.
- Give drug samples to each patient, periodically, to show you're concerned about their health-care costs.

- Give children some inexpensive gift such as a balloon, or let them pick something from a grab bag.
- Form an "I Like My Doctor Club" and invite children to join, giving them official armbands, decals, and membership cards. Each card can also serve as an immunization record.
- Call patients about the results of their tests. A brief call to say, "Ms. Jones, there's no change or cause for alarm in your blood test," can do wonders for her morale, and for her attitude toward you and your practice. But telling her, "I'll call you if anything is wrong," can create anxiety. How would you like to wait two days, three days, a week, and only then begin to relax because the doctor *didn't* call? That's an inhuman way to treat human beings. If her bill arrives after the test, but before she knows the result, the patient may feel cheated. No news is not good news. Not when your life may depend on it.
- Call patients, especially those with significant problems, one or two days after a visit, just to make sure they're feeling better. Preferably *you* should do it. If necessary, however, it can be done by a conscientious nurse.
- Keep a detailed record of all medications prescribed for each patient, so when one calls and asks for "the same thing you gave me last year," you'll know what it was.
- Talk with patients about things they're interested in.
- Select a Practice Patient Panel to meet with you quarterly and discuss their perceptions of your practice and of how you're handling their problems.

For many doctors, and for most of those in primary care, the majority of future customers will come on referral from current patients. Tailor your services and your office environment to satisfy their requests as much as possible. Never hesitate to reward or congratulate them on a job well done. Show an interest in their lives, not just their illnesses. Your rewards will be great.

Goal 2: Meet the documented needs of your patients.

Strategy: Review your latest patient survey (see Appendix D), list all the stated needs, and devise specific marketing strategies to meet them. Appendix G reviews the results of a patient survey and presents a marketing plan with strategies.

Generating New Patients _____ If you want your practice to grow, you'll also have to show those who don't know about you what you have to offer.

Goal: Develop means to make you, your services, and your practice better known.

Strategies:

■ Hold an open house for your patients and their friends. The occasion can be any change within your practice, such as introducing a partner, offering a new service, or opening a new office.

■ Offer free "get acquainted" visits for potential patients to just come by and meet you.

■ Place your practice brochure or newsletter in the local Welcome Wagon package, including a coupon for a free blood-pressure check or initial office visit.

■ Set up free blood-pressure screenings at industrial plants, retirement homes, civic meetings, or community gatherings.

■ Offer and promote free diabetes tests.

■ Support civic events by placing health messages under your name in the programs.

■ Sponsor a Little League or church sports team.

■ Send personal thank you notes to all physicians who have referred patients to you.

■ Send small gifts to show appreciation to referring physicians at holiday time.

■ Send a personalized letter (use a word processor, if possible) to any member of a patient's family who doesn't currently come to you.

■ Give copies of your newsletter to civic groups that may have an interest in a health topic it addresses.

■ If a patient tells you about a friend who's ill, send the friend health-education material that might be helpful.

The strategies you use are limited only by your imagination, so long as they're ethical and in good taste. But always remember to tell potential patients that they should return to the physicians they're already seeing. When you do, you'll be amazed at how many don't have their own physicians.

PHYSICIAN ADVERTISING
Though the AMA has changed its code to allow you to advertise, the ultimate responsibility lies with you and with each individual doctor. What you do must be based on the prevailing mood within your immediate medical community. In some parts of the country, the question is not whether you *should* advertise but *how much* you should spend. Competitive pressure, rather than inherent desire, often serves as the stimulant to advertise.

In the Miami area, for example, almost all bars are down. With ophthalmologists leading the way, a veritable advertising explosion has taken place in newspapers, and on radio and television. Scores of doctors now have public relations consultants. At least one advertises in the Miami Herald every day, as well as on both English and Spanish language radio and television stations. In more conservative areas, however, *any* advertising is considered grounds for being brought before an ethics board.

For our purposes, we'll proceed on the premise that you've resolved the ethics question and decided to try advertising. Even if you've decided not to use it, we can help you understand the strategies of those who do.

The two basic kinds of health-care promotion are:

1. *Generic*, or institutional advertising, used to promote a specialty, a health-care issue, or a philosophy of delivery.
2. *Individual* advertising, used to promote a specific physician, group, or delivery system.

Generic Advertising

This is an effective way to advance the concept of a traditional delivery system or a specialty in general. Let's assume that all the individual practicing psychiatrists within a community join together and pay for a message in the local paper. The ad emphasizes the importance of mental health, with the tag line: "Brought to you by the physicians of the Barrett County Psychiatric Association."

This sort of ad can accomplish health-educational goals by asking, for example, "Have you had your blood pressure checked recently?" The Academy of Pediatrics has done an excellent job of using advertising to educate the public on many issues, including immunization and car seat belts. Each message ends: "Brought to you by the American Academy of Pediatrics." A public service is fulfilled, and the public can't help but associate their local pediatrician with the message and the concern it reflects.

Generic Ad Strategies. A number of primary-care physicians in a southern community are concerned about the influx of freestanding clinics that advertise heavily. The physicians have seen a decline in their patient loads and have decided to include advertising in their marketing plan.

Goal 1: Devise an ethical ad campaign to help protect the individual physician's share of the market.

Strategies:

- Analyze the competition's services to see how they differ from those of individual physicians and groups in the community.
- List the strengths and weaknesses of the competition and compare them with ours.
- Develop copy and media priorities for an ethical campaign that points out the advantages of an ongoing relationship with one's personal physician.

Caution: Reactive advertising is often counterproductive. A campaign that lashes out at alternative delivery systems may be seen by the public as an attempt to "run the competition out of town." However, if you have strengths that your rivals obviously don't have, you might direct your copy to those points without mentioning names.

The primary-care physicians did just that. They pointed out that they provided a personal physician, available 24 hours a day, every day. They also noted that an ongoing relationship with one physician is far better than sporadic visits with a changing array of doctors. They ended their copy with, "Brought to you by the physicians of Smallville," and placed the ad in the local newspaper and on selected billboards. After several months, they saw a slow but steady return of their prior patient loads.

Goal 2: Provide a mechanism whereby everyone in the community can find his or her own doctor.

Strategy: The medical society places ads with a number to call if someone doesn't have a doctor. The number can be that of the society, which can then provide each caller with the names of physicians who are accepting new patients.

Figure 13-A
PROMOTION MEETS NEED

Patient Needs	Marketing Strategies
Clear Explanations	Doctor-Patient Communications
Health-Care Information	Practice Brochure
	Health Newsletters
	Educational Brochures
	Audiovisual Aids
Community Awareness	Public Speaking
	Volunteer Work
	Media Involvement
	Educational Lectures
	Ethical Advertising

Individual Advertising

When you pay for a message specifically intended to promote your own practice, you're doing the kind of advertising that most draws cries of "unethical behavior."

Individual Ad Strategies. You've just opened your practice in an urban area. You're having a tough time getting started because most of the other physicians are older and have a lock on available patients. You decide to try to build your practice through advertising.

Goal: Devise an ethical advertising campaign that will appeal to potential patients.

Strategies:
- Discover the wants and needs of potential patients *(see Fig. 13-A).*
- Develop a list of the strengths and weaknesses of competitors.
- Compare that list with the strengths and weaknesses of my practice.
- Develop ethical copy for ads that will point out the advantages of my practice over the competitors', without specifically mentioning them *(see Fig. 13-B).*
- Find the channel or form of media with the best cost per thousand persons reached.
- Initiate my ad campaign.
- Monitor new patients to find out how they learned about my practice, and why they chose it.
- Determine cost per patient entering the practice over a six-month period.

Ad Content

It's difficult to begin an advertising campaign, especially if you're the first to do so in your community. The decision mustn't be taken lightly. Even if it's done ethically, you may get some backlash simply because some people view any physician advertising as unethical.

A key to advertising is to tailor the copy to the one you're trying to reach. That means picking the proper media, evaluating both the exposure you'll get and the cost. If you begin an ad campaign without regard to copy, channel, or cost, you'll likely end it without achieving your goals.

To reach your desired patients and established goals, the AMA suggests that your ads include your:

- Education.
- Fees and how they're set.
- Payment and credit policies.

Figure 13-B

GENERAL AND URGENT MEDICAL CARE

At Your Convenience

- No Appointment Necessary
- Open 7 Days a Week, Holidays Too!
- 8 AM to 10 PM
- Medical Doctor Always on Duty
- Lab and X-ray Results in Minutes
- Low Cost

Medical Care for Your Routine Medical Problems

- Flu, Colds, Coughs, Sore Throats
- Fevers, Headaches, Infections
- Sprains, Fractures, Cuts
- Other Minor Illnesses and Injuries

Free Blood Pressure Check Anytime

- Workers' Compensation and Champus Claims Accepted

CARE FOR YOU PHYSICIANS
No Appointment Needed
8:00 AM — 10:00 PM

20 W. Juniper #103   Gilbert   892-6301

In our travels across the country, we've asked many doctors what they consider acceptable information in an ad. The opinions differ with the doctors' ages, the younger being more liberal. Here's their consensus of what belongs in an ad for a medical practice:

- Name.
- Type of specialty, with a simple explanation of what the specialty means.
- Board certification.
- Location.
- Hours of operation.
- Specific services offered.

When an ethical advertisement would be considered acceptable to a majority of those we asked, also varied, with the following being generally acceptable:

- Opening a practice.
- Changing location.
- Adding a partner.
- Starting a new service.

Ad Channels. Several channels of advertising may be used. Each has its own unique target markets, cost, advantages, and disadvantages. The media you choose will depend on whether you're in a large or small community, and on the amount of money you wish to spend. Here are your potential channels:

- *Yellow Pages:* Display and/or "in column" ads beyond the standard phone number listing.
- Newspapers: Don't sell weekly or county papers short; they're less expensive than dailies and have a wide variety of readers.
- Billboards: Especially in larger cities, but they're expensive.
- Widely distributed weekly shopping guides.
- Welcome Wagon flyers.
- Civic and community magazines.
- Radio: Less expensive than TV, and reaches a large but specifically targeted market; choose the station according to its demographic appeal.
- Television: Most costly, but reaches very large numbers with considerable impact.

Advertising services are also available whereby, for a fixed sum ranging up from $500 a year, you're listed in the company's files. Generic ads in your specialty are then placed in print and electronic media throughout the country with an 800 phone number. When a prospective patient in your area calls the number, he or she is immediately referred to you.

Some doctors, particularly in large urban areas with intense competition, are now employing public relations firms and spending large sums of money on advertising. A Denver company, for example, offers a package of 24 television commercials in your specialty, with your name, address, and phone number mentioned at the beginning and end of the copy. You're guaranteed an exclusive for your specialty in your area. But it costs $45,000.

We're not advocating the use of any of these media. If you decide to advertise, however, make sure you research the channels you choose in terms of numbers and types of people reached versus the expense.

And above all, examine the ethics of the media and its acceptance in terms of taste.

Summary
You don't need to use all the techniques suggested in this chapter. Your challenge is to find those that will fit into the philosophy of your practice, and that will maximize your marketing campaign. Just keep an open mind and proceed with deliberation and caution, letting your own good sense govern your decisions.

CHAPTER 14

Keeping patients once you have them

Listen to this not-so-hypothetical new patient. Is he talking about your practice?

"I'm the guy who sits in a restaurant and patiently waits while the waitress does everything but take my order. I also go in a department store and stand quietly waiting while the sales-clerks finish their chitchat. And I'm the one who goes to your office, Doc, and waits and waits and waits from 45 minutes to an hour or more past my appointment time.

"You might say I'm the 'good guy.' But do you know who else I am? I'm the one who never comes back. It gives me some grim amusement to hear of your spending thousands of dollars for new equipment and continuing education, and to see you spending more money on sharp marketing techniques to get people such as me into your office, when there were lots of us there in the first place. All you had to do to keep us was to have given a little service and shown a little courtesy."

That's what this chapter is all about—strategies and techniques for hanging on to your patients. We feel that the battle of the future will be focused just as much on retaining current patients as on gaining new ones.

POST-PURCHASE
COGNITIVE DISSONANCE
The unbearably pretentious title of this section looks like something dreamed up by the wedding of a Madison Avenue copy writer to a snobbish medical academic. Post-purchase cognitive dissonance: PPCD, for short.

That doesn't help at all, so let's put it in plain English. It simply means being unhappy with something you've bought. Or, to carry it a bit further, it means being so unhappy that you never purchase the same product again.

We've all had that experience. You spend a lot of time deciding on a new car, and after having kicked a hundred tires, you decide to buy a unique automobile, the Mark III Annihilator, guaranteed to run away from anything on four wheels. But within a week, you begin hearing rattles, bangs, moans, and screeches you never dreamed could come from an internal combustion engine. In the first six months, the Mark III spends more time in the repair shop than it does in your driveway. In disgust, you get rid of it. Are you ever likely to buy another car from that manufacturer? Of course not. You've come down with a case of terminal post-purchase cognitive dissonance.

At the moment of purchase, or entry into a practice, consumer satisfaction is typically at an all-time high. Once the purchase has been completed, however, satisfaction may begin to decline, and consumers may wonder if they made the right choice *(see Fig. 14-A)*. Therefore, to maintain a high level of satisfaction, you must immediately use ethical techniques to reassure patients that coming to you was a good decision.

Figure 14-A
WHY CUSTOMERS ARE LOST

Some — Die
Move Away

Many — Change to Competitors

Most — Are Dissatisfied With Product/Service
Perceived Indifference of the Producer/Server

Let's look at a medical example of PPCD: Immunization. You give the patient a shot for protection against a particular illness. Since that protection will eventually wear off, you give routine booster shots. If properly scheduled, they'll give lifelong protection. Likewise, if booster shots of marketing techniques are properly timed, they can give you lifelong patients.

You should begin administering your marketing boosters as soon as a patient enters your practice. Give the first shot at your first encounter, before any apprehension or dissatisfaction can set in. Once it does, immunization is useless. PPCD will come on as a complication, and you'll lose the patient to another doctor.

QUALITY AND CARE
RETAIN PATIENTS
Most consumers don't stop buying your product because they've found something better. Rather, they stop because of their experiences with you. You can prevent much of such migration by using three patient-retention strategies:

1. Provide an undiminishing quality product.
2. Keep patient care in mind and practice.
3. Take action to counter dropout.

A quality product encompasses much more than your technical expertise. Here's a quick review of the things that matter:

■ Your staff's handling of patients.
■ Your staff's attitude toward patients.
■ Your attitude toward patients.
■ The time patients wait for you.
■ The time you spend with patients.
■ The completeness of your service.
■ The overall office environment.

The Fear of Loss:
Yours and Theirs
It takes no genius to recognize that all your marketing efforts will be for naught if the patients you attract don't stay. And since your best referral source is a satisfied patient, it's going to pay you to keep them happy. Never take a patient for granted.

The last time you went to the dentist, or to a lawyer, weren't you a little apprehensive? You were in a new world where someone else was in control. That's how your patients feel. They're afraid that their encounter with you might uncover something that could seriously affect their ability to make a living, or to enjoy their lives. And, naturally

Figure 14-B
THE MATH OF SATISFACTION

+4 = Consumers who are completely satisfied with a service or product tell four people about their positive experiences.

−9 = Consumers tell nine people about their negative experiences.

enough, they're anxious about potential pain and the costs of their treatment. It's your job to counter and minimize those fears.

**Gain Four Patients,
Or Lose Nine?** ————————— Statistically, every patient who has a good experience with your practice will tell at least four people about it. That means four potential patients. But every one who has a bad experience with you will tell about nine people. That's nine who will not see you when they need a doctor. Bad news not only travels fast; it reaches more people. So even if you have two satisfied customers for every dissatisfied one, you still won't break even in terms of referrals. Clearly, you can't afford to think, "The customer be damned. I practice medicine; I don't coddle people." *(See Fig. 14-B)*

**Keep Your Practice
From Getting Sick** ————————— Practices fall ill just as people do. Developing strategies to retain patients is the preventive medicine of your planning. You have to keep your practice healthy, rather than waiting for it to come down with something potentially fatal. To find which techniques work, think first about the major reasons patients will leave you.

Counter Patient Anxiety ————————— At a recent seminar, one of the participants expressed puzzlement at the anxiety displayed by some of his patients. We asked if there was any service he received that made him apprehensive. He thought for a moment, and then, with a sheepish grin, said, "Getting my car fixed. Any time my car breaks down, I go up the wall."

"Why?"

"Because I don't know anything about cars, except where to put the gas. I'm always afraid the mechanic will take advantage of me because I've no way to judge whether he's a con artist, or an honest man—or whether he's honest, but incompetent."

That's just how many new patients feel about you as their doctor. They have no way to decide whether your services are needed, are priced correctly, or will even help them. So the more information you can impart to help them make their decision, the more comfortable they'll feel with your services.

The major cause of patient anxiety is innocence. (That's the same as ignorance, but it sounds a lot better.) They are innocent of your true worth. The more they learn about you and your practice, the more their fears will be calmed. Consider the following ways to win patient confidence:

Goal 1: Inform current and potential patients about the technical aspects of your practice.

Strategies:

- Develop a brochure clearly explaining your practice and financial policies, and the services you provide.
- Make sure all patients get copies of the brochure, and mail them to new patients in advance of their first appointments.
- In initial interviews with patients, give them time to ask questions about the practice and about you—preferably at no charge.
- Offer a free visit to any potential patient, and spend time discussing the philosophy of your practice.
- Instruct your staff to warmly welcome new patients and offer them a tour of the facilities.

Goal 2: Spend more time informing patients about their health and illnesses.

Strategies:

- Take time during patients' first visits to discuss both your view of health care and *theirs*. Include such things as preventive medicine, the need for routine physicals, and your willingness to have them participate in their own health-care decisions.
- Make sure patients understand: (a) what's wrong with them; (b) how you've come to your conclusions; (c) how the illness may affect their jobs, lives, and families; (d) treatments you may prescribe; and (e) how you're going to follow up on their care.
- Give written instructions explaining everything you've said. (Average people forget about 75 percent of what's communicated to them orally.)
- Develop your own and your staff's communication skills. Pay special attention to listening, so that everyone in your practice becomes a dynamic, two-way communicator.

■ At the end of each session, be sure to ask if the patient understands what you've said, and whether he or she has any questions. Have your staff do the same at checkout time.

Head Off Dissatisfaction

In any business, medicine included, unhappy customers tend to retaliate. When dealing with consumer goods, a dissatisfied customer may take the product back, complain to the management, or, in extreme cases, bring suit. If patients don't like what you've sold them, they may choose not to come to you again, elect to spread the bad news about you to friends and acquaintances, or sue. The first two choices—if carried out by enough disgruntled customers—can destroy a practice; the last one can destroy a career.

In an extensive study conducted in a western state, the causes of patient dissatisfaction fell into three categories: lack of communication with the physician and staff, desire for more health-related information, and failure of the doctor to involve the patient in health-care decisions. Here are some ways to counter such complaints:

Goal 1: Improve communication between you, patients, and staff.

Strategy: Candidly review your own and your staff's communication skills. Every negative experience can be changed into a positive one, if you make the effort.

Goal 2: Meet the need for more and better health-related information.

Strategy: Review the skills and innovations necessary to provide health information to current and potential patients. Talking with a patient just once isn't enough. You must use your communication skills in every encounter.

Goal 3: Let patients be active partners in making decisions about their health care.

Strategies:
■ Inform patients of all the facts involved in your diagnosis.
■ Tell them what you plan to do, and why.
■ Explain procedures, and any alternative methods of treatment in ways they can understand.
■ Always ask for their input, their feelings.
■ Sign "contracts of partnership" with patients, if they agree to abide by the decisions that are made. This, of course, is not a legal document, but it's a psychological prompter to the idea that a partnership exists and that it entails responsibilities on both sides.

Many physicians cling to the idea that the patient should do it because the doctor says do it. They're reluctant to give up their sense of superiority in the delivery of health care. At times that attitude must be taken, especially in very complex matters of life or death. But that's certainly not the situation in most encounters with patients.

Patients don't necessarily want to *make* decisions. They do want the facts. Physicians who deny patients access to the information necessary to make medical decisions will find their patients feeling manipulated. More importantly, they may find themselves in the middle of a malpractice suit based on failure to provide information to allow the patient the right of informed consent.

Take an Exit Survey

When patients leave a practice for any reason other than moving out of the area, many physicians simply forget about them. But that's like the coach of a losing team not trying to learn anything from the loss. Coaches normally spend a lot of time reviewing game films so they can correct their mistakes in time for the next game.

Physicians should do the same when they lose patients. The way to do it is by taking a leaf from TV network news. On election day, to find out how people voted, the networks conduct exit polls. Use a variation; call it the exit interview. Of all the surveys we've discussed, this one is probably the most difficult to do, and to evaluate. Both physician and about-to-be former patient may be uncomfortable discussing the reasons for parting, especially if there has been personal conflict. In such circumstances, how can you be sure exiting patients will give you their real reasons?

One good tactic is to assure them that, even though they're leaving, you're still concerned about their health and would like to help them find another doctor. Make sure they understand you're available until they do connect with another physician.

Face to face is usually best, but you can also phone the patient, or have a staff member make the call. If even that seems too difficult, at least write and ask for a reply. Remember, you're trying to identify specific reasons for the change. The sample questions in Figure 14-C should help you organize your exit survey. Those are the essential questions, but you may want to ask many others.

Keep this in mind: If only one or two patients suggest a particular reason for leaving, you might be skeptical. But if many patients zero in on particular problems, you've identified some practice and marketing weaknesses that must be corrected.

Figure 14-C
SAMPLE PATIENT EXIT SURVEY

Why Are You Leaving Our Practice?

1. Are you moving:
   - ☐ Outside the city?
   - ☐ Within the city but closer to a more accessible medical practice?

2. Has your employer required you to leave us because of the way your health-care benefits are now covered?
   - ☐ If yes, to which type of practice are you transferring your health care?
   - ☐ HMO
   - ☐ PPO
   - ☐ Discount doctor

3. Did you find our location inconvenient:
   - ☐ To home?
   - ☐ To hospital?
   - ☐ For other reasons? Please specify: _____

4. Were you dissatisfied with our:
   - ☐ Staff?
   - ☐ Doctor?
   - ☐ Services?
   - ☐ Costs?
   - ☐ Billing?
   - ☐ Not accepting Medicare?
   - ☐ Not accepting Medicaid?

5. Did you feel we were lacking in:
   - ☐ Quality in our medical care?
   - ☐ Involving you in health decisions?
   - ☐ Information that you needed?
   - ☐ Health education that you wanted?
   - ☐ Other ways? Please specify: _____

Summary _____ We've agreed that post-purchase cognitive dissonance is a pompous term. But patient dissatisfaction grabs you where you live. It can lead to dropouts and damage to your best referral source—your patients. You've got to keep them happy, especially now that so many competitors are out to get them.

PART IV

MARKETING APPLICATIONS AND TRENDS

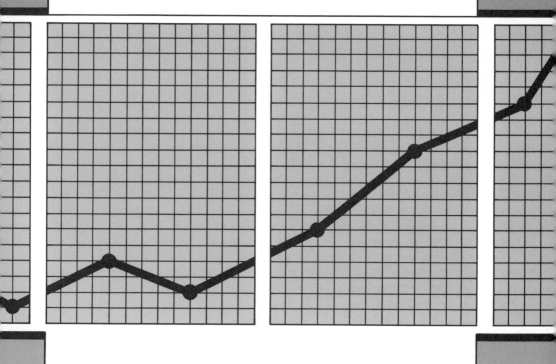

CHAPTER 15

Marketing can make you a better doctor

Can the same techniques we've been using to build practices also be used to improve the quality of care delivered? They certainly can. And that's what makes the subject of clinical-services marketing perhaps the most exciting aspect of this book. Imagine providing better health care by doing those things that improve your economic condition.

Marketing is a way to first analyze, and then systematize, the services you offer, the way you provide them, and the patients who receive them *(see Fig. 15-A)*. The entire process should result in helping the sick to get well, the chronically ill to gain a better quality of life, and the healthy to stay that way. In short, it should bring a higher standard of care to all patients. Skeptical? Think of it this way:

Suppose you find ways to help hypertensives comply better with their medication regimens, provide better care to diabetics, and get patients more involved in their own care. Wouldn't you then be able to say that you have dramatically improved the quality of your service?

Yes, marketing strategies can help you achieve all that—and more. But if *your* marketing program isn't geared to achieving those goals, it may not be beneficial to you, your practice, or your patients—no matter how many customers it attracts.

Figure 15-A
MARKETING STEPS

1. Identify Goals
2. Identify Target Markets
3. Analyze Market Wants and Needs
4. Develop Market Strategies
5. Evaluate Effectiveness

FIVE STEPS TO
MARKET GOOD MEDICINE Here's how the five steps of the marketing process can be used to improve the quality of care you deliver:

Step 1. Set Goals We've discussed the goals you should establish for your whole practice. But what about the goals for a particular service offered within the practice? Suppose you're in primary care and spend a lot of time treating hypertensives. One goal might be to improve their medication compliance. If you're an orthopedist, you might want to achieve better rehabilitation regimen compliance by post-op hip or knee patients. Such goals directly affect the quality of care delivered, and ultimately affect the overall health of the patients.

Consider these examples of clinical services goals for a number of different practices:

Specialty	Improvement Goal
Pediatrics	Immunization Compliance
Internal Medicine	Hypertension Compliance
Family Practice	Diabetes Control
Obstetrics	Prenatal Compliance
Allergies	Asthma Control
Surgery	Post-op Compliance

As indicated earlier, you must be realistic about how much can be accomplished in terms of the number of patients helped in each area. Unless your objectives are attainable, you're setting yourself up for disappointments.

Step 2. Identify Targets

Every patient should be treated as the unique individual he or she is. But don't forget that numbers of individuals often have special common needs. By using market-segmentation principles, such people can be identified, and special services can be designed to meet their needs.

Go through your charts, separating patients according to specific problems: hypertension, diabetes, glaucoma, allergy, pregnancy. Some examples of how this can be done within selected specialties:

Specialty	Market Segment
Pediatrics	Well Babies
	Chronic Ear Infections
	Allergic Children
	Asthmatics
	Orthopedic Problems
Family Practice	Hypertensives
	Diabetics
	COPD
	Sick Children
	Upper Respiratory Infection
Cardiology	Post-MI
	Coronary Bypasses
	Arrhythmias
	Chronic Congestive Heart Failure
Pulmonary	COPD
	Asthmatics
	Industrial Lung Diseases
	Pulmonary Fibrosis
Endocrinology	Diabetics
	Thyroid Disorders
	Adrenal Disorders
Dermatology	Chronic Dermatitis
	Skin Cancer
	Allergic Dermatitis
Orthopedics	Knee Problems
	Sports Medicine
	Arthritis
	Joint Injuries

Surgery	Cholecystectomies
	Gastrectomies
	Colostomies
	Post-op Care

Dividing your patients in this manner, you can quite readily identify what's necessary to appeal to each target market.

Step 3. Identify Needs

With the same methods you used to zero in on what needed to be done to retain and attract patients, you can satisfy the clinical needs of the various market segments you've singled out. For example:

Your treatment of a hypertensive satisfies his or her need for controlled blood pressure. But you must also think about the patient's other needs that can, if satisfied, lead to better compliance, and thus, to better long-term health. Think along the same lines for diabetics, whose needs are different from those of hernia patients, whose needs are different from those of children with chronic ear infection, whose needs are different from those of children with asthma. The list is virtually endless.

They all have in common the need and want for quality medical care. Beyond that, however, your job is to identify their other needs and wants.

The research required to improve the quality of care you deliver falls into three categories: clinical information to improve your expertise in a particular area, information that can lead to detection of a particular problem, and information that can help you fulfill the needs and wants of patients with that problem.

It's one thing to assume that physicians have the expertise to provide quality services for a particular problem. Yet many doctors dismiss the last two areas of research—detection of disease, and satisfaction of patients' needs—as unnecessary.

At one of our recent seminars, we asked what information was important in providing better care for hypertensives. "All I have to know about the hypertensive is how to diagnose, and what medication to use," was the comment of one physician. Many others agreed.

That answer completely ignores how patients perceive a product. A look into the marketing research available on hypertension quickly reveals that clinical expertise may not be enough.

Fact: 25 percent of hypertensive patients are not keeping their pressure under control, despite the clinical expertise of their doctors.

Fact: 50 percent of hypertensives, given quality care, drop out of the treatment program within the first year.

In other words, no matter how good you are, technically, an average of one out of every two of your hypertensive patients will either be out of control or out of your treatment program within a year. The figures dramatically reflect the problem of noncompliance in our health-care system. So, since the purely clinical approach works only half the time, is noncompliance the fault of the patient, the doctor, or are both to blame?

Brian Haynes and the team of doctors who researched and wrote *Compliance in Health Care*, found seven keys to noncompliance:

1. Poor physician-patient communication.
2. Unclear instructions by the physician.
3. Problems with office personnel.
4. Lack of patient knowledge (education).
5. Patient dissatisfaction.
6. Low patient motivation.
7. Insufficient supervision.[1]

So, just as communication, education, dissatisfaction, attitude, and staff are the major elements affecting your patient load, we now see those same factors cropping up in the area of noncompliance.

Here's how to organize a clinical-services marketing problem list that identifies what various patient types may require in addition to your technical medical care.

Clinical Problem	Marketing Problem	Patient Need
Hypertension	Compliance	Communication Education Supervision Staff's Support Doctor's Support
Diabetes	Detection	Communication Public Education Screening Convenience Reduced Fear
	Control	Communication Self-Education Motivation Affordability Follow-up

Clinical-service lists can be developed for almost any health-care problem. Each list will be different. Each will be aimed at a different target market. And each will present its own problems in detection, treatment, and compliance. But the outcome for all of them will be better detection and improved compliance, major factors in creating a higher quality of care.

Step 4. Meet the Needs
Once you've targeted a market problem—say, noncompliance—identified patients with the problem, and determined their needs in relation to the clinical services you can provide, you're ready to develop strategies to meet those needs. You will accomplish this through your clinical services marketing mix.

At this point, a review of Chapters 9 through 13 will remind you of the strategies for practice development that can also improve your clinical services.

Product. In marketing clinical services, the way you "package" your product has a direct impact on how your patients perceive it. You must pay attention to the surroundings in which your product is delivered, the interpersonal skills used to deliver it, and the use of staff in its delivery.

Price. Chapter 10 offers a detailed look at the influence the cost of your services has on the patient. Pricing from the clinical-service viewpoint gives rise to additional questions: How often does the cost of a specific service keep patients from accepting it? How often will a patient refuse a service, or become noncompliant, because the cost is too high?

No one really has the answers. Yet "cost is no doubt an important barrier to compliance for many patients."[1] That puts the physician in a bind. You can't, of course, discount services to every patient on the premise that the cost may prohibit some from accepting care. So you must look at innovative marketing tools that can provide the services in a cost-effective manner that doesn't destroy your bottom line.

Several marketing techniques can help give patients positive perceptions of cost, and in many instances won't even adversely affect the financial well-being of your practice. Providing free screening tests for glaucoma, diabetes, or hypertension will cost you something. But you'll be more than compensated by the new patients who join your practice after first being attracted by the free tests.

The nonmonetary cost of a service is especially important in clinical-services marketing. A big reason for noncompliance is fear of a particular disease. Consider the situation of a 40-year-old man with severe heart problems. Regardless of how high the price of his tests may be, it doesn't compare to the price he pays in fear and apprehension: He's afraid he'll lose his job, be unable to pay his bills, lose his sexual function, perhaps die. That personal price must be taken into account when dealing with a clinical service. Such marketing techniques as improved communications, involvement with family members, and intensive education will play a major role in the ultimate success of the treatment plan.

Place/Accessibility/Distribution. Physicians provide most of their clinical services in their offices or hospitals. How often does a treatment plan fail because the clinical service isn't accessible or convenient to the patient? How many hypertensives drop out of care because they see no reason to miss work when they feel good, just to have their blood pressure checked?

Convenience is important to the ultimate success of any clinical service. The highest quality care will be ignored by many patients if it's difficult to get to. So consider offering early morning hours to give patients blood-pressure checks on their way to work. Alternatively, stay open later at night. Every doctor can find some way to make office hours more convenient for patients.

Promotion/Communication. It's all well and good to have an excellent practice, competitively priced, and accessible. But what good will it do sick people who need you if no one knows about it? Your knowledge of glaucoma may be excellent, but if your patients, current and potential, know nothing about the importance of detection, you may have very few to treat. Clinical-services marketing uses promotional and communication tools to educate patients and detect disease. You should have the skills we talked about in Chapter 7 to enhance public education so that more patients will realize the importance of early detection and treatment.

Promotional tools can be used to inform your current and potential patients (the general public), about smoking, exercise, diet, high blood pressure, and cancer prevention. The same tools can be used to inform patients, through your newsletter, about the importance of compliance in hypertension, diabetes, and breast self-examination.

Enhanced communication will improve each patient's understanding of his or her disease and treatment plan. When patients are informed about the importance of certain clinical services, they're more likely to use them. And when they better understand their diseases, they're also more likely to be compliant.

Step 5. Evaluate Effects

A successful clinical-services marketing plan requires that your approach to a specific clinical problem be periodically re-evaluated to determine its success, and the patient's compliance with it. Of all the marketing steps, this one has perhaps the greatest effect on compliance with clinical services. How often does a physician diagnose a disease, initiate a treatment plan, and then forget to check on patient acceptance of the plan? Ask any doctor treating hypertension what the compliance rate is, and more often than not the answer will be, "I don't know."

When physicians institute such programs as periodic chart reviews, patient profiles oriented to clinical services, patient notebooks for specialty services, or patient-recall systems, the compliance rates increase. All of the above are ethical marketing tools. All help patients' overall perceptions of the practice, and enhance the implementation and success of any clinical service. And they also give the physicians a solid fix on their compliance rates.

A WINNING PLAN

How well can a plan work? Appendix H presents a complete clinical-services marketing plan to deal with the delivery of hypertensive care. Does it work? Before implementing that plan, the physician co-author of this book found that his hypertensive compliance rate was around 30 percent—about the national average. Within a year of applying the marketing approach, the compliance rate climbed past 70 percent. The result is a higher quality of hypertensive care to more compliant patients. Patient, physician, and practice are all winners—an example of successful clinical services marketing.

Summary

Our emphasis is on *clinical*. The marketing approach simply makes clinical services more patient oriented and increases patient acceptance. When physicians use their best clinical skills, design a service tailored to meet the needs of patients with specific diseases, help patients learn about and use the clinical services, and continue to monitor the effectiveness of the treatment plan, the end result is a healthier practice.

Reference

1. Haynes BR, et al: *Compliance in Health Care*, Baltimore: Johns Hopkins University Press, 1979.

CHAPTER 16

The computer can win you patients

Once we only played games on them. Now we bank, shop, pay bills, and do our taxes with the aid of computers. Almost every business uses them, and many couldn't function without them. The health-care industry hasn't escaped their influence.

In a recent survey conducted by the American Academy of Family Physicians (AAFP), close to 20 percent of the responding physicians said they use computers in their offices, and another 72 percent said they're interested in getting started.[1] The computer is clearly on its way to becoming a standard piece of physicians' office equipment.

Before you take the plunge, you must decide what hardware and software you need. You'd be wise to seek out a local computer consultant who is familiar with medical office computer systems. And when you do, be sure to talk with some of the doctors for whom the consultant has set up systems to find out how well they work.

Medical practices have used computers primarily for recording and billing their accounts receivable, and for processing insurance forms. Software for clinical records has not yet made much of an inroad, but that may change.

Computer programs have helped many practices become more efficient. Yet their maximum usefulness hasn't been exploited. A well-written medical practice program can also perform many functions in marketing. For purposes of this discussion, let's consider the marketing implications of the computer in the following areas:

1. Marketing Research
2. Demographic Analysis
3. Tracking
   a. Target Markets
   b. Patient Generation
   c. Patient Retention
   d. Personal Goals
   e. Practice Goals
4. Strategic Planning
5. Clinical-Services Marketing
6. Combating Noncompliance
7. Review of Marketing Plan

We'll tackle each area in terms of the ultimate goal of the software system, the marketing function performed, the requirements of the system, and the marketing benefits. You should choose software that has the capacity for as many of those programs as possible, as well as the capacity to use the types of modalities that are likely to be developed in the near future.

MARKETING RESEARCH

This is the most difficult task for beginners. It involves the collection of data that accurately represents your practice. For example: What's the average age of your patients? What's the profile of a typical patient in terms of sex, marital status, economic status, frequency of visits?

In making a survey, how do you select patients who will give you a cross section? Most doctors don't have such data readily available and would have to spend hours or days going through their records. A program set up to do it could put the data at your fingertips in minutes. To set up and activate such a system you must follow through on two connected goals.

Patient Profile Goal

Collect, file, and be able to retrieve patient profiles representative of the practice. Profiles should be based on age, sex, family size, marital status, demographic characteristics, geographic distribution, diseases, and frequency of encounters.

Marketing Function: Store and retrieve data that can be used to conduct marketing research.

System Requirements:
- Produce a representative profile of patients to be used for a practice audit.
- Generate a mailing list of those patients.
- Print survey letters to send to patients, or to be given to them when they come to the office. The system could even flag patients' names so that your secretary can distribute surveys when appointments are scheduled.

Marketing Benefits: The information obtained from this research can be used as the basis for periodic practice audits. The system can also generate mailing lists and address labels.

Problem Breakdown Goal Break down the numbers and types of medical problems encountered in your practice. Examples: How many patients have hypertension? Mitral valve prolapse? Degenerative arthritis? Those and other clinical questions should be stored in the system and be easily retrievable on an aggregate-practice or individual-patient basis.

Marketing Function: Use data based on clinical diagnoses in developing marketing strategies to improve the quality of care and patient compliance.

System Requirements: Record the major diagnosis for each patient. This information should be updated at each visit.

Marketing Benefits: If you can rapidly identify patients' specific diagnoses, you can use patient-recall techniques, and also pull records on those patients to monitor their compliance.

PRACTICE DEMOGRAPHICS Demographic data can help determine trends in your practice. Where are your current patients located? Where do your new patients come from? Is there a difference in the demographic distribution of your old and new patients? Are there requests to transfer patient records? If yes, where are they sent? Have any patterns emerged that can help identify competitors? Those questions can be answered quickly if your computer has access to demographic data.

Demographic Analysis Goal

Obtain a demographic analysis of your practice based on information about age, sex, number in family, working parents, and location within the community.

Marketing Function: Assess your current practice population and pinpoint locations of strength and weakness.

System Requirements: Design your system to assign a code to patients (families) that will identify them demographically. Readily accessible data should include a summary of numbers and percentages of the total patient population living in various sections. This information should be updated periodically so that emerging trends can be easily spotted.

Marketing Benefits: Information obtained from your demographic analysis can form the basis for a practice assessment. This information can then be updated to track growth trends within the practice.

TRACKING

Suppose you set a goal for your practice of, say, five new patients per week. How will you know if and when you reach your objective? With only one or two goals, it would be easy. But if you're trying to track several preset goals, computer recall is much more effective. A computer can print out the number of new patients entering your practice each week, and tell you where they come from. You can then review the data and measure the success of your goals, and you can make adjustments in tactics as needed.

Practice Growth Goal

Track predetermined areas within the practice to compare actual trends with desired growth.

Marketing Function: Assess short- and long-term marketing goals in such areas as practice growth per unit of time, ages and major diseases of new patients, and income/overhead growth.

System Requirements: Track various characteristics and match them with these five preset and preprogrammed marketing goals:
   Target Markets. Track the demographic characteristics of new patients. If you've set the goal of serving, say, more geriatric patients, a program can be set up to track the number of such patients seen.
   Patient Generation. Track and produce updated figures on the number of new patients entering the practice each week, month, and year.

Patient Retention. Track the number of patients leaving the practice and compare with preset estimates of practice decline.

Personal Goals. Track certain personal goals, such as: number of patients seen per hour, day, week; number of days off; and amount of time spent with each patient.

Practice Goals. Track marketing goals of the whole practice, such as: growth, utilization of new services, and income/expense ratio.

Marketing Benefits: A basic need in marketing is setting goals for practice growth, personal wants and needs, and overall practice satisfaction. Each area should be tracked and compared with your overall marketing goals. This comparison enables you to detect flaws in specific goals, as well as to confirm success in others.

STRATEGIC PLANNING
How can you effectively change your current product unless you know its strengths and weaknesses? How can you price competitively without knowing the effects of your current pricing patterns? Your overall effectiveness will be improved when you're able to plan marketing strategy based on solid information from past and present experiences.

Service Development Goal
Record, store, and retrieve for analysis, data that can be used in your marketing strategies.

Marketing Function: Use practice data to implement and improve marketing strategies.

System Requirements:
- Measure current and proposed services. When a new service is incorporated into the practice, the system should allow you to track utilization on a weekly, monthly, or yearly basis. Data included are the number of procedures (tests) performed and the number of patients seen for a particular clinical service.
- Combine old and new services on a spreadsheet to analyze cost and evaluate cost-effectiveness.
- Break down names and numbers of patients with certain diseases, using such coding as HTN for hypertension.
- Record significant-risk factors for each patient. Examples: Records of patients with family histories of heart disease, high blood pressure, diabetes, or breast cancer should be flagged, and lists of those patients maintained.

- Retrieve data on the types of services patients receive outside your practice. Family physicians, for example, should record which women get gynecological care elsewhere, and which parents take their children to someone else for pediatric care.
- Identify which members of particular families go elsewhere for health care, and for what specific reasons.
- Record the reasons for each referral outside the practice, and track referral physicians and patterns.
- Identify patients who will most benefit from a particular treatment, such as Pneumovax or a flu shot. This can be done, for example, by calling up the names of all patients over 65 who have heart disease or diabetes.
- Enhance the patient's perception of an efficient, modern, and caring practice.

Marketing Benefits: You should be able to evaluate utilization and cost-effectiveness of both old and new services. In this way, poorly utilized services can be dropped, and services that are not cost-effective can be re-evaluated. The ability to spot patients who go elsewhere for services you offer gives you an excellent marketing opportunity. Identifying "at risk" patients also gives you valuable information that can be used in patient education and as motivation for preventive medicine.

Accessibility Goal
Collect, store, and retrieve data on the convenience and use of the current location(s) of the practice.

Marketing Function: Retrieve data that will allow assessment of the marketing benefits and drawbacks of the practice location(s).

System Requirements:
- Evaluate the use, cost, and income from each place of service (office, satellite, nursing home, etc.), to determine cost-effectiveness.
- Draw from demographic data to evaluate the strategic placement of the practice.
- Track patient use of other providers, such as freestanding emergency centers and emergency rooms.

Marketing Benefits: You should be able to collect and analyze data on how patients regard the practice location. That data will note the use of other provider locations by patients, and compare it with the patients' locations. This will help identify current and future competitive systems.

Cost/Price Goal

Measure the overhead/price/income ratios of the practice.

Marketing Function: Evaluate cost and translate this into more competitive pricing, lower overhead, and improved cost/income ratios.

System Requirements:
- Identify factors affecting your practice overhead.
- Analyze the cost-effectiveness of a particular service.
- Identify cost-effective services of the practice so they can be given maximum exposure among the patient population.
- Present price-per-service data that will allow comparisons between your charges and current pricing practices within the community. That data can be obtained and programmed into the computer every six months.
- Utilize all data for maximum cost-effectiveness for both patient and practice.

Marketing Benefits: A practice should provide competitive pricing while allowing for a fair profit. Collection and analysis of pricing data can improve the effectiveness of your cost-containment techniques, and provide competitive pricing.

Promotion/Outreach Goal

Store and retrieve data for use with your ethical marketing techniques.

Marketing Function: Refine ethical marketing techniques, such as a practice newsletter, a recall system, and a thank-you program to expand current and potential patients' knowledge of your practice.

System Requirements:
- Generate a mailing list of all patients in the practice, all patients seen in the past two years, and all patients seen within the past year, including addresses and labels for newsletters.
- Generate recall reminders to patients about upcoming physicals and other appointments.
- Produce health-surveillance and health-maintenance notices for all patients with family histories of particular disorders, such as hypertension, diabetes, heart disease, or breast cancer. Print letters every six months notifying them of the importance of certain checks or examinations, such as yearly blood sugar tests for diabetes.

- Print abstracts of patient records that can be given to them when they travel.
- List all referral physicians (and patients), and print personalized letters, at least quarterly, thanking them for the referrals.
- Keep an up-to-date record of industrial-medicine patients, including their evaluations, treatments, and recommendations for return to work. Send that information periodically to all employers. (This will, of course, be supplemental to workers' compensation reports.) This marketing tool presents an excellent opportunity to demonstrate your interest in employees and employers.
- Identify demographic trends within your practice and show geographic trends of practice growth that can be used in marketing.
- Generate a current immunization record for each pediatric patient.
- List all patients who might need a flu shot, the Pneumovax, or other specialized immunization, and print letters notifying them of the availability of those shots.
- Track all new patients, their uses of your services, and follow-ups, and write letters welcoming them to your practice and inviting their comments.
- Write and print a quarterly newsletter.

Marketing Benefits: Medical marketing techniques are an integral part of the overall marketing strategy of any practice. A computer can store and retrieve data that will enhance your outreach efforts. Data can be used for recall, and for generating notices, bills, reminders, and letters of appreciation. The system can also help you direct your efforts to specific areas of your practice and beyond.

One of the greatest potentials the computer has is its ability to help you deliver a higher quality of care. Can you quickly draw up a list of all the patients in your practice who are at risk of developing heart disease? When it's time for flu shots, can you immediately identify the patients who need them? Computer systems can.

Clinical-Services Goal Classify all patients according to primary disease, risk factors, and health trends.

Marketing Function: Recall specific health information on patients.

System Requirements:
- List all patients with a specific disease, and mail them health-maintenance information and checkup reminders.

■ Record specific health-care data on each patient, such as: blood pressure, significant lab data, and summaries of office visits. Your recommendations can then be printed every year and made available to the patient.

■ Develop data banks for any number of diseases, and identify patients whose data bank for a particular disease is incomplete.

Marketing Benefits: State-of-the-art techniques and equipment can be programmed to enhance the quality of care you deliver.

One of our major health-care problems is the difficulty of getting patients to follow their treatment programs. Hypertensives don't take their medication, diabetics fail to follow their diets, knee-injury patients miss their physical-therapy appointments.

Are patients basically unmotivated? Or could it be that you're not spending enough time developing techniques to help them comply? Do you have the resources to identify problem patients early? A good computer system could help you combat those problems.

Compliance Goal
Identify specific patient traits and patterns to help you increase compliance.

Marketing Function: Identify noncompliant patients. Making problem patients aware that you're monitoring them motivates them to comply and reinforces their positive perception of you and your care.

System Requirements:

■ Tabulate and bring to your attention for follow-up phone calls or letters the names of patients who miss appointments.

■ Flag appointment dates of patients for whom noncompliance may mean high risk, say, those on medication for hypertension. In that simple way, missed appointments are immediately brought to your attention.

■ Recall the names of all patients with specific risk factors for periodic review of their health-maintenance records. Patients who don't keep up with specific requirements—such as annual Pap smears, mammograms, or blood sugars—can be identified, and marketing techniques instituted to bolster compliance.

Marketing Benefits: Once noncompliant patients are identified, specific marketing techniques can be used to improve overall cooperation and health.

Summary

Physicians may be the last service-oriented professionals to realize the vast potential of computers. Most of the emphasis on computer use has been in the area of financial management. It can also be used to great advantage in marketing your services.

Most systems are not all that difficult to understand and use. You can set up an infinite number of programs, bounded only by how much you are willing to expend. A wide selection of computer magazines publish roundups of available systems for educational, recreational, and business oriented software. Experienced consultants in medical office computer systems are available, and colleagues who have working computers can give you guidance.

CHAPTER 17

Marketing can help defuse malpractice threats

Unless you've been incommunicado for the past 20 years, we don't have to explain that the medical profession is in the midst of a malpractice crisis. More to the point of this chapter is how the profession has been meeting that crisis.

To a large degree, we've been looking at it from a reactive point of view; that is, our reaction to the threat of being sued has been to upgrade skills, avoid risks, have better documentation, and take other defensive measures. Practicing that kind of "defensive medicine" may be a more effective strategy for defending a malpractice suit than for preventing one. A proactive—or prophylactic—approach might serve us better.

Traditionally, we've assumed that a malpractice suit is a questioning of a doctor's clinical competence. Marketing research, however, has discovered that a good many malpractice suits involve the patient's misunderstanding of the service the doctor provided.

Why do patients misunderstand the services we provide? And why don't we understand what triggers patients to sue? Clearly, if we understand the sources of their dissatisfactions, we'll be well on the way toward finding the means to eliminate at least some of their reasons for suing.

WHY THEY SUE

All through this book we freely substitute such business terms as customer and product for your patient and the health care you provide. Our purpose is to get you thinking of yourself and your practice as components of a business that has to be marketed much like any other. But when it comes to customer satisfaction, medicine is distinctly different from other businesses.

Unlike other products, medical services deal directly with personal well-being—often in life-threatening situations. They also extend beyond the individual patient to include family and friends. Given the high expectations, involvement, and intimacy inherent in the medical-exchange process, it's easy to see why your services can result in extreme levels of either great satisfaction or bitter disappointment.

When consumers of most products are dissatisfied, they have a choice of actions. They can simply do nothing. They can grumble to their friends. They can return the offending item and demand an exchange or their money back. They can complain to the manufacturer, to government agencies, and to consumers' advocates. And in extreme cases, they can sue.

When patients are dissatisfied with medical services, they see their choice of actions as much more limited. They can't return the product because it's not tangible. Nor do they feel that complaining to you, or to anyone else, can correct the distress they feel they've suffered. Basically, they're left with a choice between doing nothing or suing. And what they do often depends on their degree of dissatisfaction.

Research studies suggest that people are less likely to complain about services than about goods. Yet they're far more likely to take drastic action over extreme dissatisfaction with a service. That may explain why many a doctor had no hint of a patient's dissatisfaction—until the patient sued.

KEEPING PATIENTS SATISFIED

It should be fairly clear at this point that the marketing strategies and skills we've discussed throughout the book can help you fend off malpractice actions. Properly applied, marketing principles will help satisfy your customers. And satisfied customers seldom sue.

Don't misunderstand. We're not trying to pretend that you can commit grievous medical errors or inflict injuries on patients and think they'll ignore them just because your office is comfortable, your staff polite, and you've been sweet. Ignore those things, however, and aggrieved patients won't think twice about suing.

Consumer orientation—thinking in terms of your patients' needs and wants—must be central to any strategic planning effort. On finding that consumer orientation topped the list of reasons why America's best businesses succeed and continue to grow, Thomas Peters and Robert Waterman, the authors of *In Search Of Excellence*, made this key point:

"Probably the most important management fundamental that is being ignored today is staying close to the customer to satisfy his or her needs and anticipate his or her wants. In too many businesses [read medical practices], the customer has become a nuisance whose unpredictable behavior interferes with normal operating procedures." [1]

That says a lot about the malpractice problem. Medicine has traditionally been service-oriented, not patient-oriented. But that doesn't mean physicians aren't interested in their patients. It does mean they've practiced more for their own satisfaction than for that of their customers. So maybe doctors can learn some principles from America's most successful enterprises.

Marketing research has identified three needs or wants that consistently characterize today's consumer. All are inversely correlated with patient dissatisfaction, and all concern what may be the most important patient perception of all—communication. Here's what patients want:

1. More Dialogue. People who are most likely to sue believe that doctors don't explain health matters adequately; they want more and better communication with the medical community. Since doctors have played a large part in creating an aura of mystery about the medical profession, it's up to them to take a doubly active role in establishing open channels of communication between themselves, patients, and others involved in their patients' care.

Doctors must make sure that both they and their patients have a clear understanding of what services are being purchased, probable costs, and probable results. That dialogue should be maintained throughout the medical-exchange process so all parties are kept current as more information becomes available. That can do a lot to give patients more realistic expectations of what can be done for them.

2. More Health Information. Those most likely to sue feel that neither the doctor nor members of the medical staff spend enough time providing health-related information. The physician, therefore, must fashion a program that allows more "quality time" with patients and their families. Specifically, the doctor must do a better job of explaining the illness, the tests, the costs, the possible course of the illness, and the probable outcome—all while being empathetic.

3. *More Involvement*. Those most likely to sue feel that doctors keep patients in the dark; they want to be more involved in their own care. Physicians rightfully believe that they should make the major decisions regarding a patient's treatment. The patient, however, must be made to feel a part of the whole approach to his or her medical problem. Patients who feel that they've been informed about their illnesses, and given reasons for the various tests and specific treatments, will feel involved in their own health care. Involved patients are automatically more satisfied patients. And satisfied patients are far less likely to think in terms of lawsuits.

HOW PATIENTS JUDGE
YOUR QUALITY
The quality of the doctor is generally thought to be the most important deterrent to malpractice. Physicians believe that if they keep up with CME, read the journals, and stay current on new technology, their patients will perceive them as quality physicians. And, as that belief would have it, patients who see their doctors as quality practitioners will never sue. Wrong!

What we're finding is that most patients have no idea of how to judge their doctor's quality. As we've noted earlier, they're more than likely to judge using surrogate perceptions that are not based on the doctor's competence, but on often distorting impressions of the physical plant, the staff, and the doctor's attitude.

The fact that you may be judged almost exclusively by the manners of the person at your reception desk, and that all your training, all your CME credits, and all your experience may not matter a whit, can be more than a little unnerving.

A doctor attending one of our seminars in Seattle responded by saying, "You mean my ultimate success depends on that 'girl' to whom I pay minimum wages?" That's right, Doctor. All other factors being equal, that "girl" could be responsible for a patient's decision to sue you. Think about it awhile. It should clear your head of some preconceived ideas and give you a whole new outlook on your profession.

The message that should come through is that everyone in your office must be involved in the marketing process. Your professional and economic success can hinge on the professionalism of your receptionist and nurses—those traditionally underpaid and overcriticized women and men.

Doctors fortunate enough to have loyal and competent staff members probably don't appreciate how many times their employees bail them out. Many doctors don't realize how often they, themselves, anger patients, and how their employees end up smoothing the ruffled feathers and massaging the hurt feelings of those patients. On the other hand, many doctors also fail to realize how often the reverse is true—how often a perfectly content patient leaves the office mad as a hornet because of something a staff member did or didn't do.

Staffers can be of immense help by anticipating needs in regard to scheduling, payments, and advice, and by playing a part in a multitude of matters pertaining to the patient's total health care. Remember the important want of patients for more health information? What better people to reinforce your efforts in this area than your staff? They're a vital link in your overall efforts to create a positive patient environment.

Summary

Viewing malpractice from the perspective of the patient puts the problem in better focus. Compliant behavior is a powerful force in the marketplace, whether consumers are buying hamburgers or health care. It's vital that we all become more consumer oriented—more attuned to the needs and wants of our patients—because patients who perceive that most of their needs and wants have been met are obviously going to be more satisfied, even if the end result isn't all they hoped for. Satisfied patients are far more likely to take this attitude: "Well, things turned out badly. But the doctor and staff did their level best and treated me very well." People who feel that way seldom sue.

Reference

1. Peters TJ, Waterman RH: *In Search of Excellence.* New York: Harper & Row, 1982.

CHAPTER 18

Marketing: Passing fad or practice fixture?

No matter where you practice medicine, you must by now have felt the tremors of dramatic and rapid change. Costs are way up. Existing and proposed government regulations threaten to strangle the life out of individual private practice. Business interests are competing fiercely with you, and so are traditional providers. Patients are reshaping the way medicine is practiced by demanding participation in their own health care, and by making more of their own—often well-informed—decisions about treatment alternatives. America's growing preoccupation with health-care economics and general fitness has led to a decline of inpatient services and an increased emphasis on preventive and outpatient care.

The major question is, "Can the individual practice of medicine become extinct?" A leader in the health-care industry recently began a seminar on marketing by saying, "If the private practitioners of this country don't wake up, we [the alternative delivery systems] will have no problems. But if they do, we might be in for a fight."

The dynamic changes taking place in today's health-care environment must be met head-on by the individual practitioner. Innovative physicians, utilizing the principles and resources of medical marketing given in this book, can and will be able to meet the current demands. But what about tomorrow? What will the future of our health-care industry be? And can today's marketing principles be applied to tomorrow's challenges?

TEN MEGATRENDS

John Naisbitt opens his best-selling book, *Megatrends*, with the following: "As a society, we have been moving from the old to the new. And we are still in motion. Caught between eras, we experience turbulence. Yet, amid the sometimes painful and uncertain present, the restructuring of America proceeds unrelentingly."[1]

The medical profession is also moving from the old to the new, and is feeling the repercussions of a turbulent environment. But after experiencing the past, and living the present, do we have any better insight into where we're going? Can we anticipate the future? More important: Can we do anything about it?

No one knows definitely what our profession's future will be like. Yet we must take a long, hard look at potential changes. We may not like what we see, but if we're to survive, we must anticipate our future. The more we learn, the better able we'll be to meet the challenges head-on.

Borrowing from Naisbitt, we see 10 megatrends *(see Fig. 18-A)* in our professional future:

1. Consumer Orientation

We are seeing the end of physician domination in the field of health care. Medicine, like most other services, will be geared to consumers' demands. Patients are taking an active and educated role in selecting medical service, basing their judgments on what they see as quality service that they can afford. The competitive medical environment of the future will have no place for the new doctor who hangs out a shingle and expects people to come in. Doctors, young and old, will be scrambling for patients. The laws of supply and demand will prevail. More than ever, marketing will be vital to the physician's survival.

2. Entrepreneurial Growth

Tomorrow's health-care industry could reach the trillion dollar level. We're now looking at the leading edge of an aggressive, marketing-oriented movement. In the future,

Figure 18-A
10 MEGATRENDS IN HEALTH CARE

1. Consumer Orientation
2. Entrepreneurial Growth
3. Vertical Integration
4. Free Market Competition
5. Big Business Domination
6. New Hospital Orientation
7. Reimbursement Control
8. Corporate Growth
9. Alternative Delivery Systems
10. Independent Practice

there will be chains of freestanding primary-care centers, ambulatory-care centers, and surgicenters. We've noted that Sears is now providing offices for dental practitioners. They're also experimenting with primary-care physicians' offices. Other major chains will certainly follow.

Stock analysts predict that one of the leading growth industries will be health care. They're not just talking about equipment, but about providers as well. Eventually, nondoctor-oriented businesses will provide a large variety of diagnostic testing, and the care, for example, for hospices, geriatrics, hypertensives—and much, much more. Many of these "futuristic" medical businesses are operating right now. Many will be staffed by nonphysician providers, perceived by patients as able to give service at much lower cost than doctors.

3. Vertical Integration
We may soon see the development of "vertically integrated systems" that will bring together under one roof, providers at all levels of health care. In exchange for sophisticated management and marketing assistance, individual practitioners would become members of larger organizations. The centers of such systems may be for-profit hospitals, HMOs, or PPOs.

Vertical systems will attempt to lock in patients for every kind of service, from one-shot emergencies to long-term care, with the individual practitioner serving as the referral doctor. Many such systems are functioning now, recruiting private practitioners in the surrounding area in large numbers. To many physicians, a vertical system will seem an acceptable alternative to the new, dog-eat-dog environment. Doctors who don't join "the system" will be locked out of the patient-referral base.

4. Free Market Competition

The future medical environment will be subject to the forces of a free market system; that is, the laws of supply and demand will be in control. In a free market system, when supply outweighs demand, consumers are in control, and the cost of the product goes down. Two main options then remain for providers:

The first is to limit their own numbers. This won't be possible in the medical field because the number of physicians can't fail to increase. There is no legal way to restrict the creation of new doctors. The other option is to develop more effective ways to compete. Again, this megatrend calls directly for use of marketing skills.

5. Big Business Domination

In 1984, Americans spent more than $360 billion on health care—almost a billion dollars a day. An increasingly large portion of this is being paid by business. Industry's investment in the health care of employees has become one of the most rapidly escalating business expenses. Chrysler, for example, has to sell 70,000 automobiles just to pay its health insurance bill. Industry will be taking a more and more active role in controlling costs, both through direct interaction with insurance carriers, providers, and workers, and through lobbying on state and federal levels.

We've already seen industry-financed HMOs and other forms of promised "cost-effective" care. If industry sees the private doctor's office as too expensive, it will tend to seek more care in megacomplexes, where medical services can be delivered in a prepaid, tightly cost-controlled environment.

Individual physicians who are deemed too costly will be hard pressed to survive. The private doctor's first "contact" with future patients may be through a business executive who comes in with a briefcase full of potential customers—if the price is right. If it isn't, he'll take his briefcase elsewhere. Private physicians who don't join may end up scrambling for patients among the wealthy, who'll be virtually the only ones left able to afford private care.

6. Hospital Diversification

Hospitals will no longer be "diagnostic and treatment hotels." Many services currently offered will be done on an outpatient basis, and hospitals will find themselves in heavier competition with each other and with their medical staff members. The community-owned facility won't be able to compete with the business know-how, economic resources, and marketing skills of the larger, for-profit organizations. The majority of hospitals will be privately owned.

Hospitals in the 1990s will be largely devoted to critical care. They'll be the final referral centers for the "vertically integrated system." Many of their current services, such as radiology, pathology, diagnostic testing, and physical therapy, will be pulled out of inpatient settings. The Health Data Institute estimates that close to 30 percent of inpatient hospital care is unnecessary and could be better provided in an outpatient setting. Future entrepreneurs will find those services easy to establish in outpatient facilities.

Hospitals will also begin to diversify. By offering potential patients more cost-effective outpatient services, they'll seek ways to lock patients into their system from cradle to grave. Hospitals will open their own primary-care centers to compete directly with local doctors. The centers will be used as referral bases for more critical inpatient care.

The newest trend for hospitals is "joint-venturing," in which two or more entities venture into a mutual sharing of physical resources, dollars, and patients. One of the most common forms: The hospital contracts directly with staff doctors, who agree to utilization review, cost-containment, and—in some cases—acceptance of discounted or prearranged fees. The hospital then contracts with area businesses, insurance companies, and even the government to bring new patients into the hospital's physician pool. In essence, the staff doctors form a PPO, and the hospital provides the PPO with patients.

To increase its patient base, a hospital may also form relationships with outlying doctors. In this type of joint venture, hospitals help doctors with their marketing, office management, and records. In exchange, the doctors guarantee to send their patients only to the affiliated hospital.

The precise direction for hospitals can't yet be predicted. But it's certain that the hospital of the 1990s will be entirely different from the hospital of today.

7. Reimbursement Control

Physicians who cling to the idea of retaining the freedom of an open-payment system are having a pipe dream. We're moving toward budgeting of care, and the age of contract medicine is well on its way. Tomorrow's health-care system will be almost totally controlled by the reimbursement system.

Diagnosis Related Grouping (DRG) has totally changed the health-care picture. This payment system is now used by the federal government to set designated fees for Medicare charges based on categories of treatment, no matter in what hospital or region of the country. Obviously, hospitals will be forced to closely monitor their doctors' utilization and cost-containment activities.

Today, the relationship between hospital and medical staff is "quietly cordial." Before long, however, tensions will begin to build because hospitals will begin to take an active stance in formulating medical policy. Hospitals will not be able to survive if physicians overutilize and overspend. So more and more, the solution will be to deny privileges to those doctors who do.

Hospital administrators will largely determine who joins the medical staff, and part of that decision will be based on the physician's proven ability to deliver cost-effective care. It doesn't take a lot of imagination to see a section of a future hospital staff admission form labeled, "Please list your charge for such-and-such procedures." If the doctor's charges are too high, privileges will be denied.

A dramatic change will take place in the independent practice of medicine when DRGs are applied to the office setting. Doctors with a high volume of Medicare patients may not be able to survive unless they use innovative ways to control costs. With practice costs soaring, the only place for cuts may be in the doctor's income. How long will doctors tolerate lower incomes before they join forces with a megagroup to help lower overhead?

"I'll not accept assignment!" has become the battle cry of a growing number of private physicians. The issue of mandatory assignment, although defeated in the 1984 Congress, will sooner or later become law. If you understand past and present trends, you can see that the legislators will have no choice.

"I'll not treat Medicare patients!" is another cry. But to stop caring for a large segment of the patient population because of bottom-line economics will threaten the survival of any doctors who try it. Many alternative-delivery systems are waiting in the wings to take over care of the ever-swelling numbers of geriatric patients.

"There will always be patients covered by other insurance carriers." True. But many of the major carriers will use the same DRG system, and many will require mandatory assignment. If these carriers find private physicians reluctant to accept prospective payment, they'll require, or at least induce, their policyholders to go elsewhere.

"Patients will never stand for these changes!" But consider the following scenario: Two of your patients, a young working couple, are covered under Company X through their employer. One day, they're told that from now on, their visits to Dr. Y will cost only $3 each. But if they continue to come to you, they'll have to pay a deductible and a copayment. Do you really think that in the economic environment of the 1990s they'll continue to come to you? They really won't.

The employees of a large Cleveland bank now have the choice of using doctors and hospitals that have a PPO contract with the bank, or using a doctor of their choice. The employee who chooses the PPO plan pays $42 a month; the employee who uses his or her longtime doctor pays $88 a month, plus a $250 deductible and 20 percent of the bills after that.

The federal government, private insurers, and employers are all going to use the reimbursement system to their advantage, and the individual physician may find the reimbursement environment too powerful to compete against.

8. Corporate Growth
In his book, *The Social Transformation of American Medicine,* Paul Starr states that physicians have escaped the corporate and bureaucratic control that characterizes almost every other aspect of American business life by channeling the development of hospitals, health insurance, and other medical institutions into forms that didn't intrude upon doctor autonomy.

He goes on to predict, however, that "the last decades of the twentieth century are likely to be a time of diminishing resources and autonomy for many physicians."[2] So unless there's a radical turnabout in economic and political policies, he concludes, the physicians of tomorrow will be quickly brought in line with the corporate structure that encompasses all other aspects of the economy.

Large corporations are rapidly becoming a central force in the health-care system. The individual doctor's loss of resources and control will come primarily from the tendency to form vertically integrated systems. Several important movements will directly influence private practitioners.

The most dramatic corporate expansion has taken place in hospital care. In 1961, there were only five consolidations of hospitals in the United States; by the early 1970s, the number had grown to 50. In 1980, a survey showed that 245 multi-hospital systems owned or managed institutions with a total of 301,894 hospital beds. Since 1968, the for-profit hospital industry has grown faster than the computer industry.

This corporate invasion brings with it an arsenal of standarized management, accounting, and marketing skills. It also introduces standardized and centralized control. In the future, decisions to admit new doctors to the medical staff may be in the hands of a corporate headquarters, not the medical staff. The "join our team—or else" philosophy may prevail, especially in light of the DRG. Doctors may be forced to accept prearranged fees or else lose admitting rights.

The corporation will select the heads of departments, establish cost-containment standards, and thus control not only the economic, but also the medical destiny of the hospital. A form of George Orwell's "Big Brother" may be realized.

The corporate structure will also bring to health care the conglomerate HMOs. In the early 1970s, all prepayment plans were locally controlled. Only the Kaiser group had expanded into a network. By 1980, the majority of HMOs were being drawn into similar networks run by such corporations as Kaiser, Blue Cross, CIGNA, and Prudential. In the future, with the withdrawal of federal start-up capital, HMOs increasingly will become part of huge corporations that have the money and expertise to attract large numbers of participating physicians and squeeze nonmembers out of the community.

9. Alternative Delivery Systems

The major change in the health-care system will be that consumers will be able to pick and choose, not just according to availability, but according to which system best satisfies their wants and needs, including price. The most popular alternatives will be HMOs, PPOs, and a plethora of nonhospital-oriented services.

The HMO alternative now attracts close to 15 million Americans, and the numbers are growing. Contrary to previous thinking, consumer research reveals that the majority of patients are as satisfied with HMO care as they were with traditional physicians.

But what about the cost of HMOs in the future? Physicians' organizations will continue to criticize them for their cost, since an HMO has enormous start-up expenses subsidized mostly by the federal government, i.e., taxes. Future HMOs, however, may be totally financed through private funds from corporations and other entrepreneurs. Many firms are committed to the HMO concept and are willing to keep the movement progressing. An example of this commitment is the Nashville-based Health America Corporation. Formed in 1980, it already owns 18 HMOs serving 400,000 members in 10 states.

Competition for patients and the growing expense of medical practice will cause many doctors to contract with such large groups and to offer their services at fixed rates in exchange for a guaranteed patient base. And employers and insurers will seek this preferred-provider arrangement more and more. New health plans, including PPOs as well as HMOs, are multiplying at astonishing rates, and will continue to be the fastest growing form of alternative delivery systems.

An increasing number of doctors will defect to prepaid care, as they tire of worrying about competition, patient load, and not being paid appropriately and promptly. As for new doctors, many will join health plans because of large education debts, fear of inadequate patient loads to provide the income to repay those debts, and fear of getting lost in the competitive marketplace.

If you don't join a PPO, you may be driven out of business. As an increasing percentage of patients are covered through their employers, the contractual relationships between industries and PPOs will grow. Industries won't be willing to let you see their employees unless some form of preset fee schedule—the heart of the PPO concept—is ageed upon.

More and more services will move out of the traditional hospital setting, and tomorrow's consumer will be able to pick and choose from a variety of services offered in a more cost-effective environment: emergency centers, surgicenters, and primary-care centers.

The home health-care industry grew from 146 approved agencies in 1976 to almost 1,000 by 1983. With the increased emphasis on earlier discharges from hospitals, it will expand even more.

A surging geriatric population and the cutbacks expected in Medicare coverage for nursing homes will provide a future for smart business people to cash in on day care for the elderly.

10. Nonprivate Practice

This chapter began with the most important question in this book: Will the individual practice of medicine become extinct? Let's ask the question in a different way: Will the individual practice of medicine survive the megatrends that are shaping the future? The answer:

Analysts predict that medicine will no longer be practiced in the traditional fee-for-service manner. Nor will it be practiced by the individual doctor acting as his or her own agent. The individual physician simply can't compete with the growing demand for the more cost-effective medicine that health-care leaders feel can be delivered only in the corporate medical world of the future.

A CALL FOR PROACTIVE CHANGE

Can individual physicians survive? We've purposefully written this chapter to alarm you—to shake you up. Although some of those trends may take years to develop, your response can be either reactive or proactive. To date, most physicians have behaved reactively to the changes confronting them.

Depressed as you may be by the trends, take heart. Doctors can survive as individual practitioners! But only if they take a long, hard look at the ways they currently practice, are willing to look at medicine and health care from the perspectives of consumers, and are willing to satisfy the wants and needs of consumers and the demands of those who pay the bills.

Can that be done? Is there a way to maintain the needed autonomy that the art of medicine demands, and still meet all the rigid demands of the new system? The authors feel the answer lies, in part, in the emerging proactive concept of medical marketing.

Summary
_____ If the concepts presented in this book are followed, the individual practitioner will at least have a fighting chance. Despite the pessimism apparent in this chapter, the future can definitely be promising for those progressive and innovative doctors who use marketing techniques. An increasing awareness of marketing by doctors and their practice managers will preserve private practice as an alternative. Remember, the same factors that challenge the future of health care in this country offer opportunities for the astute physician.

Will doctors wake up and respond to the challenges and opportunities of the changing market? Many are predicting that the doctor who continues to practice medicine as he or she chooses will soon be rare, if not extinct. But that doesn't have to be.

We agree that medicine can't be practiced as it has been, but we strongly believe that there is an alternative, a new approach to your practice. It's called medical marketing. For physicians who follow the strategies presented, the future can indeed be a win-win scenario.

We've given you the alternative. It's now up to you to take it, run with it, and use it to control your own destiny.

Good luck.

References

1. Naisbitt J: *Megatrends*. New York: Warner Books, 1982.
2. Starr P: *The Social Transformation of American Medicine*. New York: Basic Books, 1982.

APPENDIX

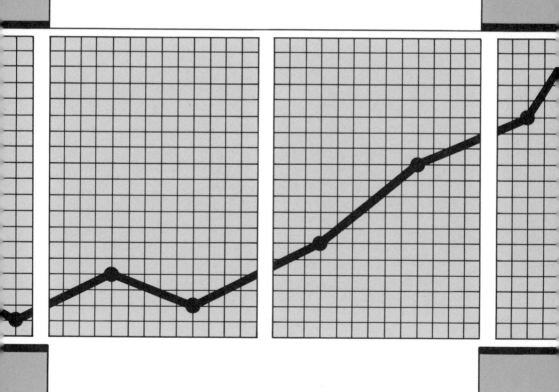

APPENDIX A

Physician self-assessment

Part A
Wants and Needs

Before an effective marketing plan can be developed and implemented, you must define exactly what you need from the practice of medicine. You can't begin a marketing plan without a direction or goal. The following outline will help you clarify your specific personal goals and give direction to your future marketing strategies.

I. PERSONAL GOALS

    A. Time Investment

        1. How many hours a week do you practice medicine?   _____

        2. How many hours a week do you want to practice?   Now? _____
               In 5 years? _____

    B. Time off for Self

        1. How many daytime hours a week do you take off?   _____

        2. How many hours more/less a week do you need for yourself?   Now? _____
               In 5 years? _____

    C. Time With Family

        1. How many daytime hours a week do you spend with your family?   _____

        2. How many daytime hours a week would you like to spend as family time?   Now? _____
               In 5 years? _____

D. Financial

    1. How much money did you earn last year after taxes? $_____

    2. How much money do you want to make?   Now? $_____

                                       In 5 years? $_____

    3. Assuming a 5% inflation rate, and a 10% yearly increase in overhead, how much will your income have to increase each year to reach your goal in 5 years? $_____

E. Retirement

    1. In how many years do you want to begin to slow down?   _____

    2. In how many years do you want to retire?   _____

II. PROFESSIONAL GOALS

A. Educational

    1. Are you satisfied with your current expertise?   Yes/No

    2. How many hours a month do you want to devote to continuing education?   _____

    3. Do you now spend that much time on continuing education?   Yes/No

    4. Are there medical interests you wish to pursue that require time out of the office?   Yes/No

    5. Will those interests provide new services that will benefit your patients and also increase practice income?   Yes/No

B. Teaching

    1. How many hours a month do you spend teaching, either in the office or at a medical school?   _____

    2. Do you want to spend more time teaching?   Yes/No

    3. If the answer is yes, do you take this into consideration when planning your practice and economic future?   Yes/No

C. Organizational Activities

    1. How many hours a month do you spend in organizational activities?   _____

2. How many hours do you want to spend? Now? _____
   In 5 years? _____

3. How many hours do those activities take away from your patient-care time? _____

4. Are you able to make up the time and money you lose? Yes/No

5. Do you plan to increase your time spent in organizational activities? Yes/No

6. If yes: By how many hours a month within 1 year?
   By how many hours a month within 5 years? _____

D. Nonmedical Activities

1. How many hours a month do you spend on nonmedical business? _____

2. Would you like to devote more time to such activities? Yes/No

3. If yes: Are your practice obligations, either patient-load or income loss, limiting your time for such activities? Yes/No

III. PERSONAL PRACTICE GOALS

A. Time

1. How many hours a day do you spend in direct patient care? _____

2. How many hours do you spend from the time you leave home until you return? _____

3. How many minutes do you average with each patient? _____

4. Are you satisfied with the amount of time you spend in direct patient care? Yes/No

5. Are you satisfied with the total time per day that you devote to your practice? Yes/No

6. Are you satisfied with the amount of time you spend with each patient? Yes/No

B. Accessibility

1. Do you feel you are accessible by phone to your patients during the day? Yes/No
   At night? Yes/No
   On weekends? Yes/No

2. Are you more or less accessible than you need to be? More/Less

3. Within the next 5 years, do you want to change your accessibility? Yes/No

4. If yes: Do you want to become more accessible, or less accessible? More/Less

C. Daily Patient Load

1. How many patients do you now see in an average day? _____

2. How many patients would you like to see? _____

3. Will a rise in your current patient load lower your enjoyment of the practice of medicine? Yes/No

4. Are you satisfied with your daily patient load? Yes/No

5. Does your current patient load satisfy your economic and practice needs? Yes/No

6. How many patients will you want/need to see per day within 5 years? _____

D. Practice Patient Load

1. Have you determined the actual numbers of patients and families in your practice? Yes/No

2. If yes: How many individual patients? _____
How many families? _____

3. If no: How many patients do you think are in your practice? _____
How many families? _____

4. Do you consider those numbers adequate? Yes/No

5. How many new patients do you average per month? _____

6. Is that the number you want? Yes/No

7. How many patients would you like to have in your practice in 5 years? _____
How many families? _____

8. That would be a change of how many patients? _____
How many families? _____

E. Patient Mixture

1. Do you know what kinds of patients (age, socioeconomic status) make up your practice now? Yes/No

2. If yes, complete the following:
   Average age _____
   Average family size _____
   Percent of families for whom you are the only primary-care physician _____

3. List in order of percentages the 5 largest age groups of patients in your practice.
   a. _____
   b. _____
   c. _____
   d. _____
   e. _____

4. List in order of frequency the 5 most prevalent disease categories you treat.
   a. _____
   b. _____
   c. _____
   d. _____
   e. _____

5. The numbers above represent the patient and disease mixture in your practice. Do those numbers (percentages) represent the overall practice you want to have?   Yes/No

6. If no: How would you like to see your practice mix change?
   In terms of average age: _____
   Treating entire family: _____
   Prevalent age groups: _____
   Prevalent diseases: _____

F. New Services

1. What are the 5 major clinical services you now offer your patients?
   a. _____
   b. _____
   c. _____
   d. _____
   e. _____

2. What other services would *you* like to offer?
   a. _____
   b. _____
   c. _____
   d. _____
   e. _____

3. What services that you do *not* offer do you feel would be beneficial to your patients?
   a. _____
   b. _____
   c. _____
   d. _____
   e. _____

4. By priority, which of the services listed in questions 2 and 3 would benefit both your patients and your practice, either immediately or in the future?
   a. _____
   b. _____
   c. _____
   d. _____
   e. _____

G. Practice Growth

(Review your answers to Part D. Practice Patient Load.)

1. Do you have enough space to efficiently handle your current patients? — Yes/No

2. Will you need more space to handle your projected patient load in 5 years? — Yes/No

3. If you had more space now, would you be able to see more patients and still maintain your present quality of care, efficiency, and cost-effectiveness? — Yes/No

4. Are you planning to expand your physical plant within the next 5 years? — Yes/No

5. If answers to 1 through 4 are yes: Have you taken those factors into consideration in your long-range planning? — Yes/No

H. Addition of Partners

1. Do you now need a new partner? — Yes/No

2. How many new partners are you planning to add within 1 year? _____
   within 5 years? _____

3. Will your current patient population support another partner? — Yes/No

4. How many new patients will you need to add per month per new partner? _____

Part B
Marketing Goals

Once analyzed, your wants and needs in Part A of this self-assessment form a personal, professional, and practice "wish list." You may choose to leave it as just that, as many physicians undoubtedly will. Those wants and needs, however, are the framework for the goals in a strategic marketing plan that can help your "wish list" come true. To see what your marketing plan goals are, use your answers in Part A to fill in the blanks in Part B.

I. PERSONAL GOALS

    A. Time Investment   Increase/decrease the time I invest in my practice by _____ hours now, and by _____ hours in 5 years.

    B. Time for Self   Increase my time off by _____ hours now, and by _____ hours within 5 years.

    C. Time with Family   Increase the time with my family each week by _____ hours now, and by _____ hours within 5 years.

    D. Financial   Increase my income by $_____ each year for the next 5 years.

    E. Retirement   Begin slowing down my practice in _____ years, and retire in _____ years.

II. PROFESSIONAL GOALS

    A. Educational   Increase my time spent yearly on CME by _____ days.

    B. Teaching   Devote _____ hours a month to teaching.

    C. Organizational   Increase/decrease my time in organizational activities by _____ hours a month.
    Maximize my effectiveness in the office and time with patients.

    D. Nonmedical   Devote more/less time to nonmedical business activities.

III. PRACTICE GOALS

A. Time

Increase/reduce my time in direct patient care by _____ hours a day.

Increase/decrease the time I spend with each patient by _____ minutes.

Increase/decrease the time I devote daily to my practice by _____ hours.

B. Accessibility

Increase/decrease my accessibility to my patients now.

Increase/decrease my accessibility to my patients within the next 5 years.

C. Daily Patient Load

Increase/decrease my average daily patient load by _____ patients.

See _____ patients a day within the next 5 years.

D. Practice Patient Load

Increase/decrease my practice by _____ patients/families a month to have the number I want in 5 years.

E. Patient Mix

Identify my current patient and disease mix and adjust it to my wants/needs.

F. New Services

Identify new services I want to offer and begin a plan to develop and infuse them in my practice.

G. Physical Space

Determine if my physical plant is large and flexible enough for current and future needs.

H. Addition of Partners

Measure the need for additional partners and the practice growth needed to support them.

APPENDIX B

Demographic analysis

Part A
Situation Factors

Physicians often spend years deciding on a community in which to set up practice, then give little time to choosing a location within that community. When well-established doctors begin to feel the pinch of competition, they examine everything about their practice—except its location. Where your practice is located can be a critical factor in its eventual success or failure. This demographic analysis will help you set important goals to incorporate into your marketing plan. It applies equally to new physicians looking for their first location, as well as to physicians who are already well-established in their communities.

I. THE COMPETITIVE ENVIRONMENT

A. Physicians

    1. How many physicians are in your current and potential practice environment?

        a. In your specialty? _____

        b. In competitive specialties? _____

        c. Others? _____

    2. Are these physicians accepting new patients?

        a. In your specialty? Yes/No

        b. In competitive specialties? Yes/No

        c. Others? Yes/No

    3. What is the average physician's age?

        a. In your specialty? _____

        b. In competitive specialties? _____

        c. Others? _____

4. How many new physicians have moved into the community practice area in the past 5 years?

    a. In your specialty?   _____

    b. In competitive specialties?   _____

    c. Others?   _____

B. Nonphysicians

1. How many nonphysician providers work independently in your community?

    a. In your specialty?   _____

    b. In competitive specialties?   _____

    c. Others?   _____

2. Are these providers in competition with you?   Yes/No

C. Hospitals

1. How many hospitals are in your community?   _____

2. Do these hospitals provide competitive outpatient services?

    a. Emergency room?   Yes/No

    b. Primary care?   Yes/No

    c. Surgery?   Yes/No

    d. Counseling?   Yes/No

    e. Others? _____ Yes/No

    _____ Yes/No

3. The following pertain to hospital policies:

    a. Is there a department for your specialty?   Yes/No

    b. Is there an "open staff" policy?   Yes/No

    c. Are privileges restricted?   Yes/No

    d. Is there a cost-containment requirement?   Yes/No

4. How many new physicians have been added to the staff within the past year?

    a. In your specialty?   _____

    b. In competitive specialties?   _____

    c. Others?   _____

D. Alternative Delivery Centers

1. Are competitive, alternative delivery centers operating in the community?   Yes/No

2. How many:

    a. Freestanding emergency centers?   _____

b. Primary-care centers? _____

c. Ambulatory surgical centers? _____

d. Diagnostic testing centers? _____

e. Industrial/workers' compensation clinics? _____

f. Others? _____

E. Alternative Delivery Systems

1. How many alternative systems function within the community?

   a. HMO _____

   b. IPA _____

   c. PPO _____

   d. Others _____

2. Are these systems a major competitive force within the community?

   a. HMO Yes/No

   b. IPA Yes/No

   c. PPO Yes/No

   d. Others Yes/No

3. Are these systems the trend in the community? Yes/No
   If yes, are they likely to affect your practice?

   a. HMO Yes/No

   b. IPA Yes/No

   c. PPO Yes/No

   d. Others Yes/No

4. Does the medical community view these systems favorably?

   a. HMO Yes/No

   b. IPA Yes/No

   c. PPO Yes/No

   d. Others Yes/No

5. Are there plans for alternative systems in the future? Yes/No

6. Do the major businesses/industries in the community require, or will they require, their employees to join these prepaid systems?

   a. HMO Yes/No

   b. IPA Yes/No

   c. PPO Yes/No

   d. Others Yes/No

II. COMMUNITY DEMOGRAPHICS

A. Population

1. What is the population of the community? _____
2. How did the number change in the past 5 years?   Increased by _____ Decreased by _____
3. Is the community considered transient? Yes/No
4. What is the population of the area from which your patients do and will come? _____
5. What is the physician-patient ratio? _____

B. Age Distribution

1. Pediatric
   a. Number and enrollment of nurseries and day-care centers? _____
   b. Number of deliveries within the community per year? _____
   c. Number and enrollment of schools? _____
2. Demographic
   a. Number of new families that moved into the community in the past year? _____
   b. Number of new houses/subdivisions? _____
   c. Number of new family apartments? _____
   d. Number of new single apartments? _____
   e. Membership growth of area churches? _____
   f. Number of new employment applications? _____
3. Geriatric
   a. Number of retirement/nursing homes? _____
   b. Presence of older established neighborhoods? Yes/No
   c. Number of families with older members living with them? _____
4. Do these age distributions correlate with the services that you provide? Yes/No

C. Economics

1. What is the percentage of unemployment in the area? _____ %
2. What are the major industries and businesses?
   a. High tech? Yes/No
   b. Heavy industry? Yes/No

c. Agriculture?   Yes/No

d. Other?   Yes/No

3. Are new businesses opening?   Yes/No

4. Are established businesses: Hiring? _____ or Laying Off? _____

5. What is the average income of your practice area? $ _____

III. LOCATION OF PRACTICE

A. Strategic Signs

1. Is your current/potential practice location situated near the patients (target markets) you want to affect in terms of:

    a. Age?   Yes/No

    b. Specialty?   Yes/No

    c. Income?   Yes/No

2. Is your location highly visible?   Yes/No

3. Is it near competitive alternative delivery systems?   Yes/No

4. Is it near physicians who will be competing with you?   Yes/No

5. Are competitive systems/physicians located between your office and your target populations?   Yes/No

6. Will your location allow practice expansion?   Yes/No

B. Accessibility

1. Is your setting near major transportation arteries?   Yes/No

2. Are you near public transportation?   Yes/No

3. Does traffic congestion make it difficult to get to you?   Yes/No

4. Do you have adequate parking and access for:

    a. Patients and staff?   Yes/No

    b. Handicapped patients?   Yes/No

    c. Ambulance loading?   Yes/No

C. Patient Convenience

1. Is your practice within 30 minutes of the majority of your patients?   Yes/No

2. Is it near the offices of most physicians to whom you refer patients?   Yes/No

3. Is it near the emergency room and other facilities you use?   Yes/No

4. Is it near other services, such as shopping malls, day-care centers, and businesses? Yes/No

5. Do your patients consider your location safe and secure? Yes/No

D. Personal Convenience

1. Is your office conveniently close to the hospitals and nursing homes you visit? Yes/No

2. Is it convenient to your residence? Yes/No

When you've done the research necessary to complete Part A, you're ready to prepare your analysis summary and draw up your demographic marketing goals in Part B.

Part B
Summary and Goals

I. THE COMPETITIVE ENVIRONMENT

A. Physicians

Situation Analysis: _____

Marketing Goal: _____

B. Nonphysicians

Situation Analysis: _____

Marketing Goal: _____

C. Hospitals

Situation Analysis: _____

Marketing Goal: _____

D. Alternative Delivery Centers

Situation Analysis: _____

Marketing Goal: _____

E. Alternative Delivery Systems

Situation Analysis: _____

Marketing Goal: _____

II. COMMUNITY DEMOGRAPHICS

A. Population

Situation Analysis: _____

Marketing Goal: _____

B. Age Distribution

Situation Analysis: _____

Marketing Goal: _____

C. Economics

Situation Analysis: _____

Marketing Goal: _____

III. LOCATION OF PRACTICE

A. Strategic Signs

Situation Analysis: _____

Marketing Goal: _____

B. Accessibility

Situation Analysis: _____

Marketing Goal: _____

C. Patient Convenience

Situation Analysis: _____

Marketing Goal: _____

D. Personal Convenience

Situation Analysis: _____

Marketing Goal: _____

APPENDIX C

Practice survey

Here are the major factors to include in a thorough survey of the effectiveness of a medical practice. Questions can be adapted to your own situation and needs, or you may choose to adopt the completed Patient Survey in Appendix D.

I. PATIENT ATTITUDES TOWARD:

A. Your Specialty

1. Do your patients understand what your specialty has to offer?
2. Do they understand the comprehensiveness of your care?

B. Your Physical Plant

1. Is your location convenient to the majority of your patients?
2. Is your waiting room comfortable and relaxing?
3. Are poor parking facilities a hindrance to your practice?

C. Front Office Personnel

1. Is your staff friendly and courteous?
2. Are calls handled promptly and courteously?
3. Do patients receive adequate help with their medical insurance claims?
4. Are your business policies (i.e., credit, cash, payment plans) adequately explained?

D. Nursing Personnel

1. Are your nurses friendly and courteous?
2. Are they sympathetic to patient suffering?
3. Do they give enough information to patients?

E. Doctor(s)

1. Do your patients feel you are courteous and friendly?

2. Do they feel you are interested in them as people as well as patients?
3. Do they feel you spend enough time with them?
4. Do they feel you give them enough information about their problems?
5. Do they feel the other doctors give them the help and information they need?

F. Waiting Time

1. Do patients feel they spend too much time in the waiting room before seeing you?
2. Do they feel they wait too long in the examining room before you see them?

G. After-Hours and Weekend Care

1. Do patients have difficulty reaching you after hours?
2. Is your answering service prompt and courteous?
3. Are the doctors prompt in returning patients' calls?
4. If other doctors are in your practice, are your patients satisfied with their service when they're on call?
5. If doctors outside your practice are in your call rotation, are your patients satisfied with the care they provide?

H. Ancillary Services and Facilities (i.e., Lab, X-ray, Emergency Room, and Hospital)

1. Do your patients resent it when you have to use other facilities?
2. Are those other facilities convenient to your patients?
3. Are their staffs courteous and helpful to your patients?
4. Do problems arise when they bill your patients?
5. Are your patients satisfied with the hospital you use?

I. Your Fees

1. Do patients consider your fees too high?
2. Do your payment policies present problems for your patients?
3. Are your patients going to other facilities for emergency care because they see them as less expensive or more convenient?

II. PATIENT NEEDS

A. Scheduling

1. Do patients have difficulty scheduling appointments convenient to them?
2. Is your staff sympathetic to patients' scheduling needs?
3. Do patients consider your office hours convenient?

B. Information

1. Do patients feel they get enough information from you and your staff about the nature and the course of their illness, and their drugs?
2. Do patients want more educational information from you?
3. Do they want a newsletter from you about their health and your services?
4. Would they use audiovisual aids if you made them available?

C. Services

1. Are patients satisfied with the range of services you offer?
2. Are there any specific services patients would like to have available in your office (i.e., pediatric care, Pap smears, minor surgery)?

III. OTHER IMPORTANT DATA

1. How were your patients referred to your practice? (By other patients? *Yellow Pages*? Local medical society? Another physician?)
2. Demographically, who are your patients?
   a. Age?
   b. Sex?
   c. Marital status?
   d. Occupation?
   e. Residence?
   f. If married, do both patient and spouse work?
   g. Do family members see other physicians? If yes, why?

Patient survey

Questionnaire Covering Letter

This is an example of the kind of covering message that should accompany your patient survey questionnaire. You should, of course, tailor it to your own situation.

Dear Patient:

We here at Center Street Family Practice Clinic want to provide you and your family with the highest quality health care possible in a comprehensive, compassionate, and cost-effective manner. To help us evaluate our effectiveness, we would like your opinions about us. Your answers and suggestions on the following questionnaire will help us continue to improve the health care we provide you and your family. So won't you please take a few moments to give us this important information?

Thank you,

Dr. *John Dole* and Staff

Questionnaire

This is a patient survey questionnaire designed for a family practice. You can easily adapt it to your own practice. Answers are provided to show how one patient responded.

I. ABOUT YOURSELF

Age: *42*   Name (optional): *MARILYN GREEN*

Sex: *F*

Address: *47 Oak Street, city*

Marital Status: Single _____ Married _X_ Widow(er) _____

Name and Age of Spouse: _Gregory (44)_

Names and Ages of Children: _Dawn (11)   Scott (8)_

Occupation: Yours _Data Processor_ Spouse _Teacher_

Education: Yours _Master's_ Spouse _Master's_

Household Income: _$48,000_

Best Times for Appointments: _Evening or Saturday_

1. Are we the main source of health care for your family?　　　　　　　　　　　　　　Yes___ No_X_

2. If members of your family are seeing other physicians, please tell us who and why.

   Spouse _____

   Children _Both children go to a pediatrician_

   Other _Mother lives with us but goes to her old Dr._

II. OUR SPECIALTY AND SERVICES

3. Do you feel you understand the specialty of our practice?　　　　　　　　　　　　　Yes_X_ No___

4. Do you believe you are aware of all the services we offer?　　　　　　　　　　　　　Yes___ No_X_

III. PHYSICAL PLANT

5. Is the location of our office convenient?　　　Yes_X_ No___

6. Do you find our waiting room comfortable?　　Yes_X_ No___

7. Do you feel relaxed in the waiting room?　　　Yes_X_ No___

8. Are our parking facilities adequate?　　　　　Yes_X_ No___

9. Do you have to pay to park when you come to see us?　　　　　　　　　　　　　　Yes_X_ No___

10. If yes, is this a hindrance to receiving your care here?　　　　　　　　　　　　　Yes___ No_X_

11. What changes would you make in the physical aspects of our office?

    None

IV. FRONT OFFICE PERSONNEL

12. Do you find our front office personnel (secretary, receptionist):

Friendly? Yes _X_ No____
Courteous? Yes _X_ No____

13. Do you find our business personnel (office manager, bookkeeper):

Friendly? Yes _X_ No____
Courteous? Yes _X_ No____

14. Are your phone calls handled in a prompt, courteous manner?

Yes _X_ No____

15. Are you receiving adequate help with your insurance?

Yes _X_ No____

16. If you need help with your insurance, can we help?

Yes _X_ No____

Need extra copies of bill.

17. Have you received a copy of our business policies?

Yes____ No _X_

18. Have our payment and billing policies been explained to your satisfaction?

Yes____ No _X_

19. Do our payment and billing policies create difficulties for you?

Yes____ No _X_

V. NURSES

20. Do you find our nurses:

Friendly? Yes _X_ No____
Courteous? Yes _X_ No____

21. Do you feel our nurses are sympathetic to your illness?

Yes _X_ No____

22. Do our nurses give you enough information about their part in your care, such as telling you what your weight and blood pressure are?

Yes _X_ No____

VI. DOCTORS

23. Do you find the doctor(s):

Friendly? Yes _X_ No____
Courteous? Yes _X_ No____

24. Does the doctor tell you enough about your illness?

Yes____ No _X_

25. Do you feel the doctor is interested in you as a person?

Yes _X_ No____

26. Does the doctor spend enough time with you?   Yes___ No _X_

27. Does the doctor give you enough health-care information, such as booklets on diet, exercise, and smoking?   Yes___ No _X_

28. Do you feel the doctor is interested in your health?   Yes _X_ No___

VII. WAITING TIME

29. Is your wait too long in the reception area before you are called to see the doctor?   Yes _X_ No___

30. Do you have to wait too long in the examination room before the doctor sees you?   Yes___ No _X_

VIII. AFTER-HOURS AND WEEKEND CARE

31. Do you have difficulty reaching us after hours?   Yes___ No _X_

32. Do you know the number for our answering service?   Yes _X_ No___

33. Is our answering service prompt and courteous?   Yes _X_ No___

34. Do our doctors promptly return your calls?   Yes _X_ No___

35. If you see a doctor in this practice other than your regular doctor, are you as satisfied with the care you receive?   Yes _X_ No___

36. If doctors other than those in this practice share after-hours calls with us, are you satisfied with the care they provide?   Yes _X_ No___

IX. PHONE CALLS

37. Are your phone calls to the doctors during the day returned promptly?   Yes _X_ No___

38. Do you mind if the nurses handle some of your calls?   Yes___ No _X_

X. ANCILLARY SERVICES

39. Do you find it inconvenient to go someplace else for certain X-rays or lab tests?   Yes___ No _X_

40. Do you find the staff at these other facilities:
Friendly?   Yes _X_ No___
Courteous?   Yes _X_ No___
If no, at which facilities? _____

41. Is the emergency room we use convenient?   Yes____ No _X_
    If no, which one would be more convenient? _Southside_

42. Do you find separate billing by these other
    facilities inconvenient?   Yes _X_ No____

43. Are you satisfied with the hospital we use?   Yes _X_ No____

44. Is this hospital convenient for you and your
    family?   Yes _X_ No____

XI. COST OF SERVICES

45. Do you feel that our fees are: High?   Yes____ No _X_
                               Average?   Yes _X_ No____
                                  Low?   Yes____ No _X_

46. Are you familiar with our credit and billing
    policies?   Yes _X_ No____

47. Have you used other health services (such as an
    emergency clinic) because you felt it would be
    less expensive?   Yes _X_ No____
    If yes, which one(s)? _EmergiCare_

XII. SCHEDULING

48. Do you have trouble getting an appointment as
    soon as you would like?   Yes____ No _X_

49. Are our secretaries helpful in finding appoint-
    ments that meet your needs?   Yes _X_ No____

50. Are our office hours convenient for you?   Yes____ No _X_
    If no, how could we arrange our hours to best
    serve you?
    Evening and/or Saturday hours

XIII. EDUCATIONAL INFORMATION

51. Does your doctor give you enough information
    about your:
                                  Illness?   Yes _X_ No____
                              Medicine?   Yes____ No _X_
                               Health?   Yes _X_ No____

52. Would you like more educational information
    from us?   Yes _X_ No____

53. Would you accept this information from the
    nurses?   Yes _X_ No____

54. If we had audiovisual tapes available on your problem, would you use them? Yes _X_ No___

55. Would you want to get a health newsletter from us periodically? Yes _X_ No___

XIV. SERVICES OFFERED

56. Are you satisfied with the range of services provided by this practice? Yes _X_ No___

57. Do you believe you know all the services we offer? Yes___ No _X_

58. Are there any specific services that you would like to see us provide? Yes _X_ No___

Examples:
Pediatric care? Yes _X_ No___
Care for elderly? Yes _X_ No___
Minor surgery? Yes___ No___
Diet counseling? Yes___ No___
Stress reduction? Yes___ No___

Others:_____

XV. REFERRAL

59. How were you referred to this practice?
Other patients_____ Friends___ _X_ _____ Yellow Pages_____
Medical society_____ Another doctor_____ Our reputation_____
Other: _____

60. Are you satisfied enough with the care we provide to refer other people to us? Yes _X_ No___

XVI. COMMENTS

Please use the space below for any additional comments you may have.

XVII. SIGNATURE (optional) _Marilyn Green_

Data Analysis Method

STEP 1. Record the total number of Yes and No responses by question.

2. Record the percentages of both the Yes and No responses for each question. Calculate the percentages by dividing the number of Yes responses by the total number of responses. Do the same for the No responses.

3. Record the Yes and No percentages for each question (See following Tabulation Sheet).

4. Assign a marketing priority number to each question (see subsequent Data Analysis Tally, page 240) by using the following classification:

RESPONSE PERCENTAGE	PRIORITY
0 - 25	4
26 - 50	3
51 - 75	2
76 - 100	1

5. Compile lists of your marketing problems by their priorities. (See Marketing Problems and Assets Priority List, page 243).

6. Determine and list the strengths and weaknesses of your practice. (See Top Practice Strengths and Weaknesses, page 245).

7. You are now ready to develop a plan of action for each of your practice problems.

Tabulation Sheet
(500 Respondents)

Q	Yes	No	% Yes	% No	Q	Yes	No	% Yes	% No	Q	Yes	No	% Yes	% No
1.	400	100	80	20	21.	480	20	96	4	41.	100	400	20	80
2.	—	—	—	—	22.	420	80	84	16	42.	450	50	90	10
3.	350	150	70	30	23.	500	—	100	0	43.	500	—	100	0
4.	300	200	60	40	24.	100	400	20	80	44.	500	—	100	0
5.	400	100	80	20	25.	500	—	100	0	45.	—	—	—	—
6.	450	50	90	10	26.	150	350	30	70	46.	500	—	100	0
7.	450	50	90	10	27.	50	450	10	90	47.	450	50	90	10
8.	500	—	100	0	28.	500	—	100	0	48.	100	400	20	80
9.	480	20	96	4	29.	400	100	80	20	49.	450	50	90	10
10.	—	500	0	100	30.	100	400	20	80	50.	150	350	30	70
11.	—	—	—	—	31.	50	450	10	90	51.	—	—	—	—
12.	300	200	60	40	32.	400	100	80	20	52.	400	100	80	20
13.	300	200	60	40	33.	300	200	60	40	53.	400	100	80	20
14.	200	300	40	60	34.	350	150	70	30	54.	400	100	80	20
15.	350	150	70	30	35.	500	—	100	0	55.	500	—	100	0
16.	—	—	—	—	36.	500	—	100	0	56.	300	200	60	40
17.	100	400	20	80	37.	450	50	90	10	57.	400	100	80	20
18.	200	300	40	60	38.	300	200	60	40	58.	400	100	80	20
19.	400	100	80	20	39.	300	200	60	40	59.	—	—	—	—
20.	450	50	90	10	40.	400	100	80	20	60.	450	50	90	10

Data Analysis Tally

Area of Practice	Question	Issue Analyzed	Response Percentage		Marketing Priority
I. Demographics	1.	Treatment of entire family	No	20	4
II. Specialty	3.	Understanding of specialty	No	30	3
	4.	Awareness of range of services	No	40	3
III. Physical Plant	5.	Convenience of location	No	20	4
	6.	Comfort of reception area	No	10	4
	7.	Relaxing environment	No	10	4
	8.	Adequacy of parking	No	0	4
	9.	Parking charge	Yes	96	1
	10.	Parking hindrance	Yes	0	4
IV. Front Office Personnel	12.	Front office friendliness	No	40	3
		Front office courtesy	No	40	3
	13.	Business office friendliness	No	40	3
		Business office courtesy	No	40	3
	14.	Handling of phone calls	No	60	2
	15.	Help with insurance	No	30	3
	16.	Need specific help with insurance	Yes	70	2
	17.	Awareness of business policies	No	80	1
	18.	Explanation of business policies	No	60	2
	19.	Difficulty with billing policies	Yes	80	1

Area of Practice	Question	Issue Analyzed	Response Percentage		Marketing Priority
V. Nurses	20.	Friendliness of nursing staff	No	10	4
		Courtesy of nursing staff	No	10	4
	21.	Empathy of nursing staff	No	4	4
	22.	Health information provided by nurses	No	16	4
VI. Doctors	23.	Friendliness of doctors	No	0	4
		Courtesy of doctors	No	0	4
	24.	Information provided about illness	No	80	1
	25.	Interest in patients as people	No	0	4
	26.	Enough time spent with patients	No	70	3
	27.	Health information provided	No	90	1
	28.	Interest shown in health of patients	No	0	4
VII. Waiting Time	29.	Reception area time too long	Yes	80	1
	30.	Exam room wait too long	Yes	20	4
VIII. After-Hours and Weekend Care	31.	Difficulty reaching after hours	Yes	10	4
	32.	Knowledge of how to reach after hours	No	20	4
	33.	Promptness of answering service	No	40	3
	34.	Promptness of doctors returning calls	No	30	3

Area of Practice	Question	Issue Analyzed	Response Percentage		Marketing Priority
	35.	Satisfaction with partners' care	No	0	4
	36.	Satisfaction with those who share calls	No	10	4
IX. Phone Calls	37.	Promptness in returning calls	No	10	4
	38.	Nurses handling calls	Yes	60	2
X. Ancillary Services	39.	Convenience of ancillary services	Yes	60	2
	40.	Friendliness of ancillary staffs	No	20	4
		Courtesy of ancillary staffs	No	20	4
	41.	Convenience of emergency room	No	80	1
	42.	Inconvenience of separate billing	Yes	90	1
	43.	Satisfaction with hospital	No	0	4
	44.	Convenience of hospital	No	0	4
XI. Cost of Services	45.	Fees too high	Yes	20	4
	46.	Understanding of credit/billing	No	0	4
	47.	Use of other services	Yes	90	1
XII. Scheduling	48.	Scheduling problems	Yes	20	4
	49.	Assistance with scheduling	No	10	4
	50.	Convenience of office hours	No	70	2
XIII. Educational Information	51.	Desire for information on:			
		Illness	No	70	2
		Medicines	No	60	2
		Health	No	70	2

Area of Practice	Question	Issue Analyzed	Response Percentage	Marketing Priority
	52.	Desire for more educational information	Yes 80	1
	53.	Nurses as providers of health information	Yes 80	1
	54.	Audiovisual aids	Yes 80	1
	55.	Newsletter	Yes 100	. 1
XIV. Services Offered	56.	Satisfaction with services	No 0	4
	57.	Awareness of present services	No 20	4
	58.	Desire for specific services:	Yes 80	1
		Pediatrics	Yes 70	2
		Geriatrics	Yes 60	2
		Minor surgery	Yes 40	3
		Diet counseling	Yes 50	3
		Stress reduction	Yes 10	4
XV. Referral	59.	Referral by %:		
		Friends	10	
		Patients	70	
		Yellow Pages	0	
		Medical society	5	
		Doctors	15	
		Reputation	0	
	60.	Satisfaction with practice	No 10	4

Marketing Problems and Assets Priority List

(Patient problems to address)

Have to pay for parking
Not aware of business policies
Billing policies difficult
Doctor tell more about illness
More health-care information
Too long in reception area
Emergency room inconvenient

Separate billing inconvenient
Use less expensive services
More educational information
Would use audiovisual aids
Interested in newsletter
Offer more specific services

SECOND PRIORITY

Improve telephone promptness and courtesy
Help with insurance
Explain payment and business policies
Let nurses handle calls
Ancillary services inconvenient
Office hours inconvenient
Give more information about illness, medicine, and health
Provide pediatric services
Provide geriatric services

THIRD PRIORITY

Don't understand specialty
Not aware of range of services
Improve front office friendliness and courtesy
Improve business office friendliness and courtesy
Want more time with doctor
Faster answers to calls
Provide diet counseling
Provide minor surgical services

FOURTH PRIORITY (Practice strengths to promote)

Treatment of entire family
Convenience of location
Comfort of reception area
Relaxing environment
Adequacy of parking
Friendliness and courtesy of nursing staff
Empathy of nursing staff
Nurses providing information
Friendliness and courtesy of physicians
Interest in patients as people
Interest in the health of patients
Examining room time
Difficulty reaching after hours
Accessibility after hours
Satisfaction with partners' care
Satisfaction with those who share call
Friendliness and courtesy of ancillary staffs
Cost of care
Understand credit/billing
Scheduling appointments
Assistance with scheduling
Satisfaction with services
Awareness of services

Satisfaction with practice
Satisfaction with hospital
Convenience of hospital

Top Practice Strengths and Weaknesses

STRENGTHS TO UPHOLD

Comprehensive Services
Convenience
Adequate Parking
Staff
Physician Attitude
Accessibility
Pricing
Scheduling
Overall Satisfaction

WEAKNESSES TO ADDRESS

Paying for Parking
Physicians not Informing Patients
Inadequate Information About Policies
Inadequate Health-Care Information
Inconvenient Emergency Room
Too Much Waiting Time
Not Enough Specific Services
No Practice Newsletter

Getting out a newsletter

PRINTING

The cost of printing a 4-page patient newsletter on white stock (an 11″ × 17″ sheet, printed on both sides and folded to 8½″ × 11″) will range from $24 to $50 for 100 copies; $45 to $70 for 300; $60 to $100 for 500. Those costs will be higher if you print in two, three, or four colors, or on color stock.

Before you pick a printer or sign a contract, be sure to shop around for the best offer in both price and quality, asking all you contact to show samples of similar publications they have done. You may even be able to get a price break on a first sample issue. Also ask colleagues who have done newsletters for printers they would recommend.

DISTRIBUTING

Getting out your newsletter can be as simple as putting copies out on tables in your reception area, or as complex as presorting, addressing, labeling, bagging, and delivering them to the post office.

Hand Delivery. Getting your newsletter directly to your patients in the office is free and easy, but you'll reach only those who are currently coming to you. If you do office distribution, hand it to patients as they check in or out; don't just lay it about the office. Extra copies with a "Please take one" card may get some patients to pass copies along to families and friends.

You may want to test a sample newsletter on patients in the office, handing it to them when they come in, then asking for any comments they may have before they leave. Improvements and suggestions they may recommend can then be developed in subsequent issues.

Even if you choose office distribution of some issues or copies, also consider mailing to reach the broadest base of patients and potential patients most regularly.

Presort and Prepare Mail. If you decide to mail, you must first decide which class to use, first or third. Either way, you must presort and prepare your mailing. And that can get complicated. So to help avoid mistakes, take a sample copy of your newsletter to your local postmaster. That will help catch any addressing or labeling error before it multiplies, and will get you specific instructions on how to seal and package your pieces. While at the post office, pick up a free copy of US Postal Service Publication 113, "First-Class, Third-Class, Fourth-Class Bulk Mailings." It contains all the details you'll need, plus illustrations, for preparing and packaging your newsletter.

Presort First Class Mail. First class is the most expensive way to mail your message. Even presorted, it will cost 18¢ a piece. Is it worth it to get your message to your patients quickly? Probably not, for a general newsletter. But a special issue on a health emergency would surely be worth it. If you want to go first class, here are the basic requirements:

- You need a minimum of 500 pieces for the Presort First Class rate.
- 10 or more pieces with the same 5-digit ZIP Code must be bundled.
- 50 or more pieces with the same 3-digit ZIP code prefix must be bundled.
- Addresses outside the 5- and 3-digit groups count toward the minimum number of pieces, but don't qualify for the lower presort rate.
- Each piece must carry the words, "Presorted First Class Mail," printed or stamped as part of, or next to, the meter imprint, permit imprint, or precancelled stamp.
- For a First Class permit imprint, you must pay a $50 application fee, and an annual $50 fee if you use a permit imprint stamp and number. There is no $50 annual fee if you use a meter to stamp your mailings.

Third Class Bulk Mail. This is a much cheaper way to go: 12.5¢ per piece, or 10.1¢ for pieces with the same 5-digit ZIP Code. If you're worried about looking late or slow, just update the issue one month, mailing your April issue in March, for example. Following are the basic third-class bulk mailing requirements:

- You must have at least 200 pieces.
- 10 or more pieces with the same 5-digit ZIP Code must be bundled (the 10.1¢ a piece rate).
- Fewer than 10 pieces with the same ZIP Code also must be bundled.
- Pieces with the same 3-digit ZIP Code prefix must be put together.
- Remaining pieces with varied ZIP Codes go together in a "city" package.
- All packages must be put into a sack, each containing at least 50 pieces. You can pick up sacks and labels from the post office.
- For a bulk rate permit, you must pay a $50 application fee, plus $50 per year to maintain and use your permit number.

APPENDIX F

How to work effectively with the media

I. The Big Picture

   A. Build an effective personal rapport with the media before a public relations crisis occurs. Meet the station managers and program directors of radio and TV stations, and the editors or publishers of newspapers and try to establish credibility and rapport.

   B. Make an effort to understand the media from *their* point of view, not just yours. Remember that media people are professionals who take great pride in their responsibility to the public.

   C. Learn the editorial philosophy of your local newspapers and radio and TV stations, and what kinds of public service advertisements and announcements they carry.

   D. Don't approach the media from either a demanding or a pleading posture. Let them know you're just as interested as they are in seeing that their reading, listening, or viewing audiences receive the information necessary to make an informed, independent decision.

   E. Share your information with the media in a concise, easy-to-understand way. Media people are intelligent, but they don't have technical expertise in medicine.

   F. Localize and personalize your concerns. Smalltown, Georgia, is far more interested in what happens in Smalltown, than in Atlanta or New York.

   G. Define a profile for the audience you're dealing with: age, sex, socio-economic status, etc.

II. The Turf

   A. Plan ahead: Thoroughly familiarize yourself with the various formats used by your radio or TV station (call-in, dialogue, monologue, or interchange), and try to participate in the selection of the specific format for your presentation.

   B. Know your interviewer. Make a point of reading, listening, or viewing several of his/her interviews. Learn your interviewer's style!

C. Do your homework: Be sure you really know the facts and facets of the subject. Provide the media with concise, factual information about the issue, both pro and con. Suggest areas of discussion, or possible questions. But don't demand them.

D. Get to the station early enough to survey the turf. Request time with your interviewer so you can "get to know each other." Warm-up time is important.

E. Address the average reading or listening audience, *not* your peers. Gear your presentation to a tenth-grade level, but don't be condescending in any way.

F. Stick to the issue. Avoid being trapped in a morass of confusion. Remember that you are providing information, not saving mankind from the evils of your opposition.

G. Don't argue. On radio or TV, arguing can come across as arrogance. Express your understanding of the opponent's view, but back up your own position with facts, not rhetoric.

H. Be concise and to the point. Any answer longer than two minutes loses its impact.

PERSONAL APPEARANCE AT INTERVIEWS

"You are what you appear to be," is a superficial approach to people. Nevertheless, personal appearance is extremely important in the media. A well-planned, well-delivered presentation becomes less effective when the audience takes more interest in your appearance than in your message. Dress, mannerisms, and voice all contribute to the impression you make on an audience. Here are some helpful suggestions on how to appear to your best advantage:

I. Appearance

   A. Wear a neutral suit or dress. "Loud" or "busy" clothes will distract the audience from what you're saying.

   B. Blue is always appropriate, although most TV cameras can now compensate for white.

   C. Neutral ties look best: wide knots for large people, slimmer knots for smaller people.

   D. Don't be afraid to ask for a little makeup. TV lights will make you look washed out, especially when compared to a well made-up interviewer.

II. Body Language

   A. Get comfortable, but watch your posture.

   B. Stay still. A constantly moving guest drives the camera people crazy.

   C. Avoid excessive hand gestures.

   D. Portray warmth and confidence. A stern look may come across as cold or unfriendly. Smile, but don't overdo it.

E. Be aware of your body language at all times. It can reveal your reaction to others. For example:
1. A clinched hand may mean anger.
2. Slouching or slumping indicates a lack of confidence.
3. Always speak to the interviewer, *not* to the camera.
4. Cross your legs in the direction of the conversation. (If the interviewer is to your right, put your left leg over your right.)

III. Voice Language

A. Speak in a normal tone. Don't shout; don't hurry.
B. Warm up your voice by going through some vocal exercises before the interview. Exaggerated vowel sounds serve the purpose.
C. Don't speak in a monotone. Vary your pitch to suit the words. Change the pace of your speech to add color, or pause for added emphasis.
D. Talk conversationally, as you would to friends in your living room. This, combined with a smile, will cover a multitude of sins.
E. Speak at a tenth-grade level. Scientific rhetoric loses the point and the audience. Make your point in two minutes or less. Longer responses aren't remembered.
F. Most of all: Have Fun!

THE INTERVIEW

Most doctors fear being interviewed simply because they're unfamiliar with the basic techniques of interviewing. The most important technique is to *be prepared*. That means knowing what the interview is going to be about, and anticipating any questions you may be asked, pro and con. Write out responses to those questions to help organize your thoughts. But never read from them during the interview, because the appearance of spontaneity is very important to a successful interview. Good preparation and the following techniques can help allay many of your interview fears:

1. *The Loaded Question:* "Since all doctors make a fortune, why don't you lower your charges?

Don't be trapped. This type of question is based on a false premise. It may be the result of ignorance, or the questioner may be baiting you. Either way, point out firmly but tactfully that you do not accept the premise on which the question is based.

Your Response: "First of all, most doctors are not making fortunes."

Then go on to discuss the cost of medical care. This approach accomplishes two things. First, you've defused the negative aspects of the question. Second, you've used the question as a springboard into a controversial topic on which you can expand your views.

2. *The Irrelevant Personal Question:* "Doctor, I understand you are a member of the local country club."

Try to avoid falling into the trap of answering a personal question that is not relevant to the interview.

Your Response: "That's not really relevant to this interview, but I'll be glad to discuss it with you after the show."

The interviewer now has two choices: to simply accept your tactic and move on to another question, or to counter by saying, "But the audience is interested in how you doctors spend your money." That turns the personal question into a hostile confrontation.

3. *The Hostile Question:* "Doctor, how much money do you make?"

This is one step beyond the "irrelevant personal question." Try to keep your temper and respond calmly that the question is personal and not relevant to the topic at hand.

Your Response: "I really don't think that has any bearing on our subject. Besides, I think the audience would be more interested in my views on health care than in the details of my personal life."

If the hostile question is pursued, you have three options:

- Re-emphasize that you feel the audience is interested in health care.
- Give general data regarding the drop in the average doctor's salary in the past few years. (If you use this method, be very cautious. Make sure your facts and figures are correct.)
- Acknowledge that you feel the question is meant to put you on the spot regarding your personal life, and that you don't feel that to be the objective of the interview. Try to get the interviewer back to the medical subject.

If the interviewer persists along a hostile line, the best you can do is to break even. Here are some points to remember:

- Stay calm and confident. By refusing to get angry, you can let the interviewer "dig his own grave." You'll be the one in control of both your temper and the interview.
- Watch your body language and voice level. Controlling them will help you control your temper.
- Never threaten to leave the interview. If the interview is terminated, let the interviewer do it. That way, he or she is the one who is responsible and has to justify it.
- Survive the moment. Keep calm. If the interviewer changes to a more acceptable line of questioning, just act as though the rudeness never occurred.

4. *The Disparaging Question:* "All I read about is how doctors give illegal drugs to patients."

Don't let implied or direct criticism put you on the defensive. Dispel the criticism if it's totally false, or emphasize that while the situation does occur, it's the exception, not the rule. You can then move on to speak of peer review, ethics committees, etc.

Your Response: "There are some bad apples in every barrel, but they are rare and we are trying to clean out the ones we do have. We have ethics committees and peer review organizations to help us identify those doctors who abuse their privileges."

Never deny criticism that is based on fact. If you do, you'll lose your credibility.

5. *The Ignorant Question:* "Doctor, are brain transplants being done now?"

In this situation, try not to embarrass the interviewer. Never imply that the question shows a lack of preparation or knowledge.

Your Response: "That's a very interesting question. Although brain transplants are not being done yet, medicine has made great advances in transplanting other organs such as kidneys, livers, hearts, and even lungs."

6. *The Question That Stumps You: "The New England Journal of Medicine* recently reported a new drug that might be the cure for cancer. Can you tell us about it?"

At one time or another, every doctor has been stumped. When you're asked a question you can't answer, or aren't sure of, simply say, "I don't know." These can be the three most important words in the language, and can earn you the respect of the audience and the interviewer.

Your Response: "I don't know, but I think it is an important point. I'll look up the answer and get back to you on it."

Admitting you don't know everything is admitting you're human; looking it up indicates the question is worth pursuing and you know where to look. You win on both counts.

Marketing plan: Patient retention

MARKETING GOAL:

Reduce by 75 percent the number of patients in practice who are using or considering using alternative delivery systems.

MARKET RESEARCH:

A significant increase in the number of requests to have medical records transferred to a recently organized HMO. A patient survey revealed:

- 50% find office hours inconvenient.
- 75% of families have both husband and wife working.
- 60% want more information about their illness and the drugs used in treatment.
- 40% have difficulty reaching the doctor after hours.
- 50% have used, or would consider using, alternative delivery systems after regular office hours.

TARGET MARKET:

- Patients currently using or considering using alternative health systems.
- Families in which both husband and wife work.
- Patients who desire more time and health information.

I. PRODUCT/SERVICE

Need	Strategy
More convenient hours	Evaluate the possibility of more flexible hours.
	Leave schedule open in early morning and late afternoon so acutely ill patients can be worked in.
	Evaluate the possibility of evening and/or Saturday office hours.

Less waiting time	Review scheduling policies.
	Confer with secretary to structure more effective appointment times.
	With nursing staff, review procedure for putting patients in examining rooms.
More time with the doctor	Consider making appointments longer.
	Re-evaluate approach and conversations with patients.
	Make time with patients more productive.
More health information	Evaluate use of more educational materials.
	Make a point of explaining each drug given a patient.
	Utilize drug information handouts.
	Explain and re-explain each illness.
	Give the patient time to ask questions.
	Provide the patient with both written and oral instructions.
Better after-hours care	Give an emergency number to all patients when they see you.
	Send a newsletter to all patients explaining coverage after hours.
	Make sure the answering service is providing good service.
	Make sure the practice is covered by an available doctor at all times.

II. PRICE: MONETARY

Need	Strategy
More economical emergency care	Educate patients that ER care is more expensive in the long run.
	Provide more in-office emergency services, such as suturing.
	Distribute a patient newsletter that explains how to handle emergencies in a more cost-effective manner.

PRICE: NON-MONETARY

Need	Strategy
More understanding from you when both husband and wife work	Show you're aware that 75% of patients come from families in which both parents work, and that an office visit often means lost wages.
Less apprehension about illness	Provide more psychological support to patients.
Less fear of the effects of the illness	Explain in detail the illness, expected course of recovery, prognosis, and when the patient should be able to return to work.

III. PLACE/LOCATION

Need	Strategy
More convenient emergency care	Evaluate location of ER now being used to see if another might be more convenient for patients.

IV. PROMOTION

Need	Strategy
Better patient understanding of the illness, drugs prescribed, and course of treatment.	Offer better patient education from doctors and staff.
	Involve nursing staff in giving health information.
	Evaluate use of more educational brochures and audiovisual aids.
	Give drug information handouts.
	Provide extensive written and oral instructions.
More health-care information	Send a practice newsletter with patients' monthly statements.
	All of the above.

V. RE-EVALUATION

Need	Strategy
Periodic evaluation of marketing strategy effectiveness	Closely monitor requests for transfer of patient records.
	Talk with patients during their visits to see if they are aware of your strategies.
	Plan another patient survey in six months, and compare results.
Update of marketing problems	Evaluate new areas of concern and indicate new marketing strategies that need to be developed.

APPENDIX H

Marketing plan: Clinical services (hypertension)

MARKETING GOAL:

Improve hypertensive services and increase patient compliance by 50 percent.

MARKETING RESEARCH:

- 22% of Americans between 25 and 74 have hypertension.
- Hypertension is a major cause of death: 750,000 annually.
- Many people are unaware that they have hypertension.
- 25% of those with hypertension do not have it under control.
- Patients lack basic education about hypertension.
- 50% of those with hypertension drop out of care in the first year.
- Drug reactions and interactions cause many to stop treatment.
- Noncompliance is a major health problem.

TARGET MARKET:

- Patients in your practice with unidentified hypertension.
- Patients now under treatment for hypertension.
- Potential hypertensives, including all of those with a family history of hypertension.

I. PRODUCT/SERVICE

Need	Strategy
Better detection	Record blood pressure on each patient at each visit.
	Get staff to screen blood pressure at local retirement homes and industries.
	Flag for identification charts of all current and potential hypertensives.

Better compliance	Extend patient education.
	Confer with hypertensives and their families about high blood pressure and its dangers.
	Set and explain blood-pressure goals for your patients.
	Follow through with periodic physicals and health conferences with patients and families.
More convenient care	Schedule blood-pressure checks at convenient hours, i.e., early morning or late afternoon.
	Direct home blood-pressure monitoring.
	Send staff to retirement homes and industries periodically to offer blood-pressure checks.
	Record blood-pressure readings on all hypertensives.
More drug information	Provide extensive written and verbal information about antihypertensive medication, with special emphasis on side effects.

II. PRICE: MONETARY

Need	Strategy
More economical care for the new hypertensive	Re-evaluate need for expensive initial evaluations.
More economical follow-up care	Offer free blood-pressure checks, which should lead to better compliance and to more regular office visits, and offset your costs for the checks.
	Use drug samples, but make sure there are no side effects from new medications.
	Assist patients with medical insurance claims.

PRICE: NON-MONETARY

Need	Strategy
Reduce the high psychological cost (fear) of having high blood pressure	Counsel and reassure patients and families to relieve fears.

III. PLACE/LOCATION

Need	Strategy
More convenient care	Set flexible hours to monitor blood pressure.
	Get staff to take blood pressures.
	Give prompt service without appointment to check blood pressure.
	Send staff to check pressures in retirement homes and factories with large numbers of centralized patients.
	Open satellite offices.
	Make house calls to bedridden or severely arthritic hypertensives.
Reduced waiting time	Tighten scheduling.
Comfortable surroundings	Re-evaluate waiting and examination rooms.

IV. PROMOTION

Need	Strategy
Better understanding by hypertensive patients and their families of hypertension and need for lifelong care.	Raise patient awareness of the disease and its control.
	Increase patient family involvement in care with family conferences.
	Spend more focused time with the patient.
	Improve quality of time spent with the family.
	Distribute educational brochures.
	Use audiovisual aids to help educate patients about hypertension.
	Distribute newsletters about how to detect and handle the disease.

Need	Strategy
Greater awareness of hypertension by all patients and the public.	All of the above. Better communication with the public about hypertension. Lectures to school, civic, and church groups on hypertension. Use the electronic media to educate the public about hypertension. Send letters to all patients with a family history of hypertension, emphasizing the need for frequent blood-pressure checks.

V. PERIODIC RE-EVALUATION

Need	Strategy
Early detection of dropouts	Review charts of hypertensive patients quarterly.
Increase compliance	Review your hypertension records monthly. Identify and contact all patients who fail to keep appointments for follow-up care.

INDEX

increases in, 10-11
medical practice and, 14
quality care and, 184-185
reimbursement control and,
207-209
See also Fees
Health Care Finance
Administration, 11
Health food stores, 36, 76
Health insurance. *See* Insurance
Health maintenance
organizations (HMOs), 3
competition and, 10, 37, 156
corporations and, 210
costs and, 14
future and, 205, 210
industry and, 206
insurance and, 115, 116
Health plans, 37
Health rights movement, 76-77
Hillestad, Stephen, 126
Holistic health care movement,
76-77
Hospital Corporation of America,
11
Hospitals
competition from, 36, 37
corporate organization and, 4,
11-12, 209-210
delivery systems and, 127
future and, 206-207, 210, 211
medical practice and, 4, 11-12
referrals and, 127-128
reimbursement and, 207-208
Hours. *See* Schedules and
scheduling

Indirect delivery systems, 126,
127-128
See also Delivery systems
Individual advertising, 165
See also Advertising
Individual practice associations
(IPAs)
competition from, 37
costs and, 14
Industry
fees and, 122
future and, 206
market segmentation and, 87-88

See also Big business;
Employers
Insulin, 5
Insurance, 4
Diagnosis Related Groups and,
208
fees and, 115-117
future and, 206
health maintenance
organizations and, 210
market research and, 47
physician's role and, 121-122
Internists, 8
Interview. *See* Direct interview
IPA. *See* Individual practice
associations (IPAs)

Journals, 20, 46-47

Kaiser group, 210

Labor movement, 14
Lanzillotti, Robert F., 113
Lawyers, 4
Location
accessibility and, 128-129, 130-
131
patient needs and, 60
satellite offices, 131-132
See also Relocation
Loss of patients. *See* Patient loss;
Patient retention

Mail questionnaire, 51, 52
Malpractice, 3, 197-201
approaches to, 197
communication and, 197-198,
199-200
patient motivation in, 198
patient satisfaction and, 198-
200
quality judgements in, 200-201
Marketing, 17-26
components of, 19
conceptual model of, 24-26
future of, 203-212
malpractice and, 197-201
narrow view of, 18-19
need for, 4-5, 22-23